MW00843777

Successful Self-Dentistry
How to Avoid the Dentist Without
Ignoring Your Teeth

Copyright ©2011 by Nadine Artemis

First Published in 2011
By
Flowers Shining Everywhere Inc.
P.O. Box 369, Haliburton, Ontario
Canada K0M IS0

1ˢᵗ Edition written in June, 2011

Artemis, Nadine
Successful Self-Dentistry – How to Avoid the Dentist without Ignoring Your Teeth

ISBN: 978-0-9877073-2-1
E-Book ISBN: 978-0-9877073-0-7

This book is designed to provide helpful information and inspiration to our readers. It is sold with the understanding that the publisher is not engaged to render any type of psychological, legal, or any other kind of professional advice. This book is not meant to be used, nor should it be used, to diagnose or treat any medical condition. For diagnosis or treatment of any medical condition, consult your own physician/dentist

Cover Design & Graphics: Nadine Artemis and Robert Howard. Set in Century Gothic

Produced in Canada

"Moisten your tongue with praise, and be the spring ground waking. Let your mouth be given its gold-yellow stamen like the wild rose's.'

Sanai
11th century Persian Poet

"Self-knowledge is the beginning of wisdom, and without that self-knowledge you cannot go far. Therefore you must begin near, and search every word you speak, search every gesture, the way you talk, the way you act, the way you eat; be aware of everything without condemnation. Then in that awareness you will know what actually is and the transformation of what is, which is the beginning of liberation. Liberation is not an end. Liberation is from moment to moment in the understanding of what is."

Jiddu Krishnamurti

"Do not leave your health in your dentist's hands and assume all will be fine."

Hal Huggins, DDS

Acknowledgments

Loving appreciation to my late night tooth brushing companion, my howdy partner, Ron, who is always up for the adventure of living. To our son Leif, whose smile fills my heart with gratitude and has taught me so much about the care of children's teeth - and whose breath is so pure. Abundant thanks to my mother's earnestness about making the right choices for her children. And, I thank the friends and family that gift our life and our house guests who let me show them a better way to brush.

I acknowledge and appreciate the maverick dentists of this century who persevered through ridicule and opposition until their tooth truth practices and discoveries could find acceptance. I also want to thank Jonathan Landsman of the *Natural News Talk Hour* and Patrick Timpone of the *One Radio Network* for interviewing many of these dental mavericks and capturing the current zeitgeist of their work.

I thank my dental hygienist Pat, who, years ago, did not summon the dentist. She instead encouraged me to, "Go home and put some of those botanical oils you mix on this cavity and we shall take an x-ray next visit and see that it has evolved."

I am extraordinarily fortunate to be surrounded by a palette of plant essences that offer their gifts and allow me to help others. I am deeply thankful to the talented distillers who keep the true art of distilling the plant's quintessence alive.

I am very grateful to Keesha and our Living Libations kin, who keep everything well-oiled: Heather, Thien-Anh, Elana, Anne, Jen, Dotty, Erin, Vik, Johnny, and Ashley. I have great gratitude to all of our beloved clients who imbibe and make making Libations such a blessing.

I thank, with an everlasting toast of chaga, David Wolfe, who encouraged me to make a tooth serum with neem and Ayurvedic herbs. I send a heartfelt thank-you to the organizational force of the Longevity Now Conference team: Rebecca Gauthier, Len Foley, Camille Rose Giglio, and Lucien Gauthier for creating such a venue of leading edge revelation.

Great thanks to the proof-readers of the manuscript: Angela McGreevy, Robert Howard, Hope MacLeod, Ben Johnson and Tami Gibson, for giving me the confidence that all of the commas are in the right places. I thank Robert Howard of Orbit Creative, who graciously translates the images in my mind to graphics and photographer Barbara Stoneham for her ability to capture essence.

I present this book as a work of care and an offering of probable solutions so that you, the reader, may empower your life.

Contents

Introduction

If you are like me and were raised in contemporary North American culture, you've been told since you were a toddler about the importance of brushing your teeth and visiting the dentist twice a year. Your parents showed you how to brush (hopefully), and, if they were diligent, they may have even showed you how to floss. By the time you were a teenager you most likely had the hang of it, but you may have also experienced cavities and other dental issues anyway, especially if you had the diet of a typical teen.

What I discovered, through my research on dental self-care (having teeth, this is a subject that interests me greatly) is that we were not really set up for successful oral care as children, and the reason is simple: our parents, even our dentists, were less-than knowledgeable about how to care for and feed our teeth and gums. Even if we brushed, flossed, and went to the dentist every six months as prescribed, we still got cavities and may have even have ended up with root canals, extractions, and other invasive procedures. We did the best we could without having the whole picture.

When you became an adult and no longer had your parents to take you to the dentist's office, you may have begun creating excuses for avoiding the dental

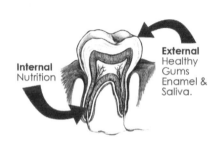

External
Healthy Gums
Enamel & Saliva.

Internal
Nutrition

chair. I made excuses to avoid the dentist; it seemed better not knowing what was going on with my mouth. Perhaps I was instinctively rebelling from the orthodontic contraptions, my nose cautious about the antiseptic ethers, my mouth recoiling from the strange taste of fluoride, metal, and foam. Yet, without wisdom to serve my rebellion, avoidance made oral entropy and, hence a trip to the dentist, inevitable.

I had also grown up with the understanding that one needs medical doctors to take care of the body and dentists to take care of the mouth. So, like many people, I developed the belief that the mouth was separate from the rest of the body. As well as becoming aware of this curious "disconnect" between the mouth and the body, I was also struck by the way Western medicine and dentistry treat the symptoms instead of the source of body imbalances. This system of treating symptoms creates a perpetual loop of appointments, medications, surgeries, scaling, bridges, crowns, and fillings that never reach the core underlying root causes of the imbalance. Treating the signs of decay, rather than the sources, may explain the statistic that 90% of sixty year olds will have 63% of their teeth missing, filled, or decayed[1].

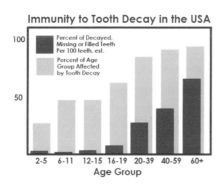

Immunity to Tooth Decay in the USA

---

[1] Statistics from Center for Disease Control: http://www.cdc.gov/MMWR/preview/mmwrhtml/ss5403a1.htm

Introduction

Thankfully, the light went bright, and I unearthed myself from this deeply embedded cultural mouth/body split. I began to understand, and feel the inherent, innate desire of the body to recalibrate and regenerate, and I knew it had to include the teeth too.

Perhaps you already have a good sense of what works in oral care. You may have already had your mercury removed, you may know about the dangers of fluoride, and you may *love* to floss. Knowing the worthiness of each tooth and being such a good oral care ambassador, naturally you are surprised when you receive reports of receding gums or a cavity on your twice-yearly visit to the dentist. *So now what?*

In this book I will share what I know about how to keep your teeth and avoid dental-stress by providing more wisdom about oral care. In truth, you *can* bypass the dentist, not because you are afraid to go, but because you understand your oral ecology and are free of active decay.

It is a matter of learning a new daily maintenance routine that involves some simple, at-home procedures that your childhood dentist knew nothing about. In the pages that follow, I will give you step-by-step instructions for creating new oral care strategies (and eliminating old ones) so you can build stronger and healthier teeth, gums, saliva, and enamel. Even if you still visit the dentist now and then, this book will help you learn how to make informed decisions about serious issues like root canals and gingivitis.

Introdution

As you read through these pages, you will become familiar with the intricate relationship between the internal and external factors that influence the health of your mouth. You will learn how to get rid of active decay, understand healthy oral ecology, and take practical steps to serve the entire body by allowing nutrition to feed your teeth. You will feel your saliva re-enamelizing your teeth, you will feel your gum pockets strengthening around each tooth, and you will wake up ready to kiss the day.

1. Your Teeth are Alive

"Even if there has been massive damage, the teeth can be repaired. In fact research tells us that teeth with early cavity damage can heal themselves once disease is eliminated from the oral environment."
Dr. Robert O. Nara, author,
"Money by the Mouthful"

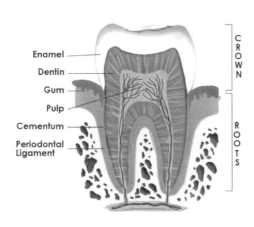

Enamel
Dentin
Gum
Pulp
Cementum
Periodontal Ligament

CROWN

ROOTS

The most exciting thing that I have discovered in my research about oral care can be summed up in one sentence: *Your teeth are alive!*

Growing up, I thought teeth were merely solid bones in my mouth, necessary for chewing and biting, set in stone, as it were. I now know that teeth are alive. Like the eyes, the limbs, and the internal organs, they respond to all the same internal factors, such as nutrition, bacteria, and trauma. Being alive, teeth can be healed, strengthened, and regenerated, meaning that the current condition of your teeth and mouth can actually *evolve*. In order to deeply understand this, it is important to understand what teeth, gums, saliva, and bacteria are all about. So, let us start with a quick overview of the internal architecture of the teeth and the mouth.

A Tooth Tour

1. The outermost layer is the **enamel**, which is constantly building up and breaking down, all day and night. Under a microscope, the enamel reveals a honeycomb-shaped crystal called a *hydroxyapatite* (a crystalline calcium phosphate). When saliva has a pH of 7, calcium and phosphate flow into the tooth enamel to build *more* crystals, which forms strong, dense enamel. When saliva is acidic, the crystals dissolve and become smaller, causing pores to form in the honeycomb pattern of the enamel. Porous teeth are susceptible to chipping, crumbling, and staining.

2. **Dentin** is the next protective mineralized layer below the enamel. Inside the dentin are microscopic tubules that, if laid out flat, stretch on for three miles! These tubules radiate outward through the dentin, from the pulp to the enamel, and contain water, fluids, and cell structures.

3. Below the dentin is the **pulp,** which contains blood vessels, cells, and nerves.

4. The roots are covered with **cementum**, which is also a mineralized collagen tissue.

5. **Gums** hold the teeth in place, upright in their sockets. The gums cover the roots and contain thousands of microscopic connective filaments that anchor the tooth to the jawbone, and the

health of these fibers is reflected in the health of your gum tissue.

In addition to these layers, each tooth also contains blood vessels, craniosacral fluid, and dentinal fluid. These fluids and their vitality connect the teeth to the body's physiological functions. Each tooth relates to different meridian paths of "Qi," or life energy as it is understood in Traditional Chinese Medicine. Qi contains invisible electric lines that run through the teeth, connecting them to a unified field of the body.

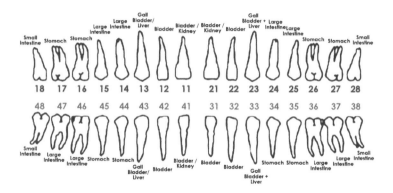

Just to get an idea of how vast and intricate each tooth is, consider the fact that one molar alone contains more than 300 meters of tubules. That is almost impossible to comprehend. Indeed, one tooth containing 300 meters of tiny tubes! Once you understand the complex creation of each tooth, it is easy to imagine how damage can be caused by dental procedures like drilling, filling, root canals, and extractions: it is like putting a chain saw to your teeth.

As an overview, remember this: the enamel is alive, the dentin inside the tooth is alive, as are the pulp, the blood vessels, the nerves, the saliva, and the gums. Teeth are more than just bone. Teeth are a mineral matrix consisting of multiple tissues of varying density and hardness. They are living things, and you must perceive the inside of your mouth as one whole living organ - a living ecological system. As such, you can see why it is so important to keep your oral ecology healthy - the gums, saliva, teeth, bone, and muscles - because they all work together within their own micro ecosystem.

Super Saliva

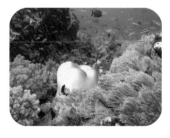

Healthy teeth exist in a sea of saliva, a sea of saline alkalinity. Imagine that your mouth is a coral reef in which your teeth are the coral, surrounded by an ocean of alkalinity. When your teeth are lubricated in healthy saliva, they are at their absolute healthiest. In this state, you can heal a lot of decay and prevent new decay from occurring.

Your saliva is extremely important to the functioning of your mouth. It contains many chemicals and enzymes that exist specifically to take care of the teeth, and it is designed to bathe the teeth all day long in a solution that has a pH of approximately 7. This is exactly what your teeth and gums need.

Saliva can re-mineralize or de-mineralize teeth. It controls bacterial flora in the mouth, prepares food for digestion, and produces certain vital hormones. The major salivary glands include the *parotid*, the *submandibular*, the *sublingual*, and the *small labial*.

Saliva is a saline solution made of enzymes, peptides, minerals, and bicarbonate. Bicarbonate ions in the saliva are linked to a healthy saliva flow rate, and a higher concentration of bicarbonate ions helps maintain the alkalinity of saliva. Saliva has a component that is similar biochemically to baking soda, which actually makes baking soda harmonious and congruent with the oral environment and a great tool for keeping your teeth clean. If saliva is too acid, it dissolves the enamel on your teeth and creates an environment that houses bacteria. The longer the mouth remains acidic the more damage is done to the enamel. Weak, porous enamel and acidic gum tissue create sensitive teeth. Furthermore, saliva that has too much alkalinity excretes excess calcium and can create calculus build up on the teeth.

The key is to allow saliva to effectively do its job. It is one of the superheroes of the mouth. When there is the beginning of oral decay, the saliva jumps into action to coat the tooth with its beautiful, healing fluid. Saliva is always active, always working to coat the teeth and help the enamel to stay strong. At night when we are sleeping, everything slows down, including the activity of the saliva, which is why bacteria grow faster at night. This is particularly true if you are on prescription drugs, if you snore, or if you sleep with your mouth open. Keep hydrated with spring water during the day, and let your saliva flow rate take care of your teeth at night.

The Gums: Turtlenecks for the Teeth

Imagine that you are wearing a very well-made turtleneck sweater that keeps you warm, cozy, and protected from the cold. Your gums do the same thing for your teeth. They wrap around each tooth like a little turtleneck; however, when there is decay or a buildup along the gum line, bacteria gets in and the gum starts pulling away from the tooth. That is what most people know as *receding gums*. Healthy gum pockets are 2-3 millimeters, but when the gum pocket starts to pull away from the teeth and the turtleneck no longer fits snugly, the gums are now sporting a crew-neck enabling bacteria to reach a portion of the tooth that 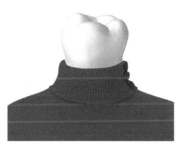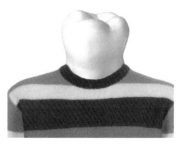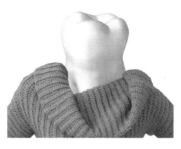 has no protective enamel. This can create sensitivity to foods and hot/cold temperatures, and can also be the beginning of decay. Mild inflammation of the gums is known as *gingivitis*. *Periodontitis* is an advanced inflammation of the gums which has been linked to premature births, irritable bowel syndrome, and heart issues. This can also happen as a result of improper brushing, poor nutrition, and other factors that are discussed throughout this book.

The gums can slowly be worn away so that the crew-neck becomes a loose-fitting cowl neck. When this happens, you can end up with exposed molars and the bone beginning to wear away. This is referred to as "bone-loss." When we experience symptoms of decay, we usually think it is the tooth that is in trouble. Yet, most of the time, it is the gums, because they are the first area to weaken. More teeth are lost to gum disease than to tooth decay. The area where the gum and the tooth meet is called the *sulcus,* and it is very, very precious. The union of the gum and the tooth is one of the most important areas to care for.

Relief comes from knowing that inflamed gums are one of the easiest issues to cure. Statistics tell us that 98% of the population has poor gum health (periodontal disease). Yet, what the population does not know is that this can be turned around, depending on your overall health, within as short a time as 24 hours! Instead of loose, dark, unhealthy gums, you can have nice bright, pink, healthy gums that do not bleed and are resistant to decay. Without surgery! Surgery may take care of the problem temporarily, however, many people find that five to ten years later their gums recede again as they fall back into old oral hygiene and nutrition habits.

Your Teeth are Alive

Remember, your gums are *alive* and they can regenerate with proper care. Even if it has been a while since you last visited the dentist and your gums are bleeding and your teeth are sensitive to cold or hot temperatures, the gum tissue is easy to heal with a few changes and daily dedication

We will go over how to make those changes in Chapter 6.

Bacteria and Decay

Your mouth is an *incubator*. It is warm and inviting: a perfect humid home for biofilm (both beneficial and deleterious bacteria) to settle in and grow. If you have a cavity, which is essentially an infection, you should think of it as an open wound. If you had an open wound on your hand, for example, you would take care of it by keeping it clean and protected, while making sure it was exposed to plenty of air circulation. It would be less than ideal to put your hand in a stagnant puddle of water or some other place that is full of bacteria. So, imagine that a cavity is an infection inside your mouth (which is exactly what it is), and that that infection can create a hole in the enamel. A cavity is a *symptom,* and the first stage is known as a *carious lesion*. When the bacteria are removed and the diet improved, a carious lesion can be halted.

Bacteria feed on food waste and then excrete waste of their own. This material combines to form biofilm (*plaque*), which builds up on the teeth, on the tongue, the cheek tissues and on the gums.

Plaque is an ideal nesting area for germs, and those germs can become well-organized *colonies* of germs, which create a perfect incubator for unwanted bacteria. Because your mouth is a living thing, these colonies of bacteria are constantly being formed and constantly being sloughed off (basically sloughing off their own excrement and dead skin cells). These cells build little colonies between the teeth and along the teeth edges. They love this environment because it helps them grow, and the result of that growth is *plaque*, which eventually becomes *tartar*, which eventually becomes *calculus*. All of these things inhibit the saliva from doing its job, which is to cover the tooth with a protective coating. When that coating cannot be applied, enamel weakens and decay begins.

That is the external story on decay, yet something that not every dentist knows is that part of the decay process is *internal* and related largely to nutrition. Our teeth are fed via the roots (like tree roots 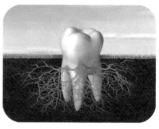 drawing up nutrients into the tree) with nutrients coming from pure food and water. Diet also plays an important role in the alkalinity of saliva: if your saliva is less than alkaline, it will eat away at your enamel. One excellent way to adjust your diet so you can alkalinize your saliva will be explored further in Chapter 5.

Because teeth are alive, they respond to caries, which is another word for the decay that starts to occur when bacteria start to damage the enamel, dentin and cementum. This can also be referred to as an enamel lesion, which means that the surface of the enamel has been compromised and a cavity is forming. A brown spot on the enamel is an indicator that this may be happening.

Because the teeth are alive, they know exactly what to do when decay is brewing. If a cavity starts to form, the dentin reacts by sending *odontoblasts* to the cavity site (the infection), where they start the healing process by laying down a secondary layer of dentin. Your saliva also responds to this. So, if you can get your saliva in the right condition, it will help to defend against a cavity!

It ranges from some little pinpoint cavities here and there all the way to a tooth that's rotted right off at the gum line, you're not going to grow a whole new crown on it. The little ones will heal, remineralize up to about two millimeters deep. What will happen in a tooth that is severely decayed is that the stump will firm up. Instead of being soft and mushy, it develops a leathery consistency. A healed tooth will remain resistant to decay as long as the oral conditions are beneficial.

Dr. Robert O. Nara, D.D.S.

The Dentin: Whiteness Comes from Within

One question that frequently comes up when discussing enamel is about how to keep teeth white. I can tell you with absolute certainty that there is no bleaching kit out there that will do the job safely and effectively, be it from the dentist or the drug store. Eventually those treatments will eat away the enamel and will cause your teeth to become even more dependent on bleaching because, as you lose enamel, your teeth will look duller. Bleaching is not recommended, ever. Furthermore, bleaching can disrupt or damage the nerve of a tooth and can cause gum recession or cause gums to shrink back. Whether over-the-counter bleaching kits or a process done at the dentist's office, all bleaches damage the enamel to some extent, ultimately making the teeth more sensitive to staining.

What you want to do is create the white from the *inside out*. So, instead of approaching it cosmetically, approach it *internally*. Enamel is transparent, and it is the dentin inside the tooth that makes it appear white. The health of the dentin is literally *reflected* in the tooth. That is the best way to improve whiteness... by allowing it to shine through. You allow it to shine through by having healthy dentin. In the following chapters, you will learn how to improve the health of your dentin, and thus, the whiteness of your teeth.

It is true that tartar and calculus build-up can discolor and create something other than pearly whites when you enjoy red wine, green smoothies, turmeric, blueberries, and other foods rich in color. This can be easily removed by polishing teeth with a mixture of baking soda and salt, which is further described in the Eight Successful Steps later on in this book. The enamel layer is actually translucent like glass. Hard, healthy, strong enamel will reflect the whiteness of the healthy dentin *inside*, so the best way to whiten your teeth is always *from within*.

2. May be Harmful if Swallowed

The Truth about Toothpaste, Toothbrushes and Mouthwash

Certainly when you were growing up everyone brushed their teeth with toothpaste, and this was exemplified as being one of the good habits required in order to have a clean mouth and prevent cavities. You may have been repeatedly advised that if you brush, floss, and go to the dentist twice a year, you will have good dental health. If you are like many people, you probably found that regardless of your good habits, you still ended up with dental problems such as cavities, gum bleeding, unpleasant breath, and more.

One of the most common diseases in North America is bleeding gums, and because it is so common, many people just ignore it by attributing it to having sensitive teeth. Bleeding gums is the body's way of responding to bacteria in the mouth. The advertising industry has done a great job of convincing us that all we need to deal with this tenderness is a product for sensitive teeth, so people go out and buy a special brand of toothpaste advertised as helping this issue, and the symptoms appear to lessen. However, the symptoms are only being masked because these types of toothpaste anesthetize the mouth without healing the sensitive teeth.

"Minty fresh" is a marketing promise we all know. Common toothpaste feels refreshing because it

16

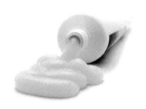 contains synthetic mint (menthol) or other flavor by-products such as cinnamon (*cinnamaldehyde*). These are not the real plant essences; they are synthetic derivatives. Eventually, understanding that many beauty care and oral care products were artificial, I switched to toothpastes from the health food store, only to realize that they too contained synthetic ingredients such as *sodium lauryl sulphate*, calcium, glycerin, and more. I also noticed that even if *did* contain herbal extracts, the extracts were not in amounts that would benefit the oral ecology in any effective way.

Foaming chemicals in your mouth while you are brushing your teeth do not create optimal oral ecology. Commercial toothpaste gives an illusion of freshness, yet it does not really remove plaque, it is the brushing that does that. It is best to be minimalist about it and use a dry toothbrush with a dab of salt, baking soda, or a *Tooth Serum*.

The chemicals used in commercial toothpaste, including many of the brands sold in health food stores, include chemicals that you do not want in your mouth, such as *glycerin*, which coats the teeth and blocks the saliva from doing its primary job of re-mineralizing the enamel. You will also find *calcium carbonate*, which is essentially chalk that is not at all good for teeth. Also, what paste would be complete without the detergent and surfactant *sodium lauryl sulfate*, which makes toothpaste foamy? This known carcinogen breaks down your skin's natural barrier, easily penetrates skin, causing bleeding gums, and allows other chemicals to penetrate by increasing skin permeability approximately 100-fold. Additionally, when combined with other chemicals, it transforms into carcinogenic nitrates and can reside in the body for five days.

Some toothpastes contain *propylene glycol,* also known as anti-freeze, which is not to be handled without gloves in a lab. Fluoride[2] in toothpaste damages gums, mottles teeth, disrupts collagen production and enzyme activity[3]. Then there's the FD&C color pigments (including coal tar derivatives that contain heavy metals and accumulate in the body), formaldehyde, Triclosan (a registered pesticide and bio-persistent chemical that destroys fragile aquatic ecosystems), artificial sweeteners, and synthetic *isopropyl alcohol.* You may also be surprised to learn that *ethanol* is the primary ingredient in most mouthwashes, even though it is known to cause approximately 36,000 cases of oral cancer[4] a year! How is it possible that carcinogens could help keep your mouth healthy? Yet when

---

[2] Fluoride in toothpaste has been found to cause acne eruptions around the corner of the mouth and chin area from the nocturnal salivary drainage of the chemicals from Fluoride toothpaste from nighttime brushing. *Fluoride Toothpaste: A Cause of Acne-Like Eruptions,* Archives of Dermatology, Saunders 1975; Volume 111; Pages 793

[3] *Fluoride the Aging Factor: How to Recognize and Avoid the Devastating Effects of Fluoride,* Dr. John Yiamouyiannis

[4] McCullough, Michael; C. S. Farah (December 2008). "The role of alcohol in oral carcinogenesis with particular reference to alcohol-containing mouthwashes."*Australian Dental Journal* **53** (4): 302–305.

people find that they have breath or gum problems, one of the first things they do is go out and get a new brand of toothpaste and a big bottle of ethanol-based mouthwash.

Can these toothpaste and mouthwash ingredients really bring decay and bleeding gums into balance?

Healthy gums provide a natural barrier against the 400-plus microorganisms entering the circulatory system. The epithelium (the *very* thin skin inside your mouth) is only one cell thick and is designed to keep toxins, bacteria, and infection from entering the body. The soft oral tissues are great at absorbing whatever comes into contact them, with approximately 90% absorption efficiency, the tiniest break or cut in the epithelium (bleeding gums) allows toxins and bacteria to enter the bloodstream quite quickly.

In the strategies shared with you in this book, you will learn how to re-enamalize your teeth by allowing the saliva to do its job while maintaining a healthy environment in your mouth. One of the most important steps in beginning this process is to stop using all commercial products and replace them with salt, baking soda, a dry brush, and botanical remedies that can begin the healing process. More on that soon.

Let's talk toothbrushes. Perhaps you have a toothbrush that is flattened out after a few months of use. Most people think this is a sign telling them that it is time to replace the toothbrush. Yet, in fact, it is telling you something quite different...that you are using way too much pressure when you brush. You want to brush lightly enough so that in six months your toothbrush looks just like it did the day you bought it, rather than a squashed version of its former self.

In the Eight Steps of Successful Self-Dentistry (Chapter 6), two types of toothbrushes are suggested: manual and electric. One type of manual brush that I have been enjoying for a decade is an ionic light-activated toothbrush. It uses light to activate its ability to ionize the saliva. Electric toothbrushes are great for learning how to change your brushing habits. They will introduce you to places in your mouth you didn't know you could reach, and I find there is very little difference between the high-priced models and the inexpensive models. If you want to buy an electric toothbrush, purchase one that has a round head so that you can reach the challenging areas behind the back and front teeth. And by the way, always use a soft-headed toothbrush.

Fun with Flossing

If you are flossing, that is great. If you are flossing with botanical tooth serums, that is even better. Flossing is something you definitely want to

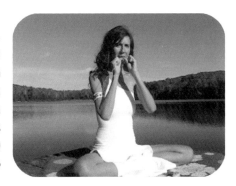

do, and the act of flossing gets revolutionized once you add *Yogi Tooth Serum* or *Healthy Gum Drops*, because these serums can reach the bacteria between the teeth. The floss gets the food out, and the essential oils send the plant molecules in to clean out the interdental plaque and bacteria.

If you have not flossed for a while, your gums may bleed. No worries. It will clear up by flossing 2-3 times a day for 2 or 3 days, *especially* if you are using the tooth serums. If you have an issue with one particular tooth and you floss that tooth with extra care, you can experience a change within a couple of days.

Evolving Habits

Because many of us find daily oral care to be a dull activity, we tend do it on autopilot. As part of developing some freshness to the daily care of your mouth, it is best to be mindful of what you are doing, and brushing teeth is a great place to start.

Instead of laying a chunk of toothpaste on a wet toothbrush while standing at the bathroom sink with the tap on and brushing with a lot of foam for 20 seconds, consider the possibility that you can brush anywhere. You can brush sitting down, or in the shower or bath...even outside in the sun or sitting at your desk. When you change your location, you will be amazed at how mindful you will become. Whenever I get the chance, my favorite place to brush my teeth is by the ocean, with the sunlight to activate my ionic tooth brush and ready-made salt water on hand for rinsing.

Here is another huge habit-changer...it is better to use a dry toothbrush than a wet one. Just stroking with a toothbrush and rinsing will remove more bacteria and plaque than using a brush with regular toothpaste. If you want to add something to your brush, try a little baking soda. The baking soda's alkalinity will be activated, which is exactly what the saliva needs. Better yet, use Tooth Serums made with essential oils, and you will get anti-fungal, antiviral, antibacterial, and lipophilic benefits that will penetrate the gums (more on essential oils in Chapter 8).

Another tip: it is less than ideal to brush your teeth right after meals. If you brush too soon after eating, the saliva will not have time to recalibrate to its slightly alkaline level of 7 pH. You can rinse with salt water to neutralize the saliva again and floss if desired.

To summarize, instead of worrying about *good* habits, welcome new intentions about the care and attention to your teeth.

3. Mad Hatters, Mavericks and Modern Dentistry

In this chapter, I am going to introduce you to several dentists who make a difference. These are the brave, out-of-the-box thinkers who have contributed to transforming the practice of dentistry. While most of their work is still not mainstream, they have paved the way for change. If you are ready to transform your oral care routines, the work of the researchers and practitioners described below will provide valuable guidelines for you.

A Visit to the Dentist in the Year 2022

As you lean back into the far-infrared chair, an osteopath attunes your cranial alignment while you and the dentist go over your latest blood work, which confirms that your recent dietary changes have resulted in your hormones and minerals reaching optimal levels. You are now ready to proceed to a brief laser cleaning.

Thank-goodness your appointment was not scheduled a decade earlier when you would have found yourself listening to *Muzak*, inhaling high ambient levels of mercury, and being exposed to radiation with routine x-rays. If a cavity was discovered, it would have been filled with silver amalgam mercury, and you would have been advised to brush with fluoride after each meal, floss (with a free sample of petroleum coated wax floss), and rinse with a synthetic antiseptic mouthwash. The hygienist would explain brushing techniques (again), and since your gum line is quickly receding, you would be scheduled for an appointment with the periodontist, who would graft skin from one part of your body to cover the deep pocket of part of the gum line.

Luckily, at your 2022 appointment, mercury fillings have been banned -- first by Sweden in 2008, and then the world -- as more patients (including dentists) were diagnosed with mercury-induced psychosis, like the Mad Hatters of the 19th century who were exposed to mercury toxicity when felting hats, which led to the ban of mercury in the hat-making industry.

Centuries ago, dental experiences included blood-letting, having good teeth pulled out to promote general health, and doses of arsenic being administered for tooth pain that often killed the nerve and then the patient. Though these procedures sound dangerous and archaic to us today, we may in the future look back at today's practices of filling teeth with toxic heavy metals, treating root infection with root canals and extracting teeth only to leave jaw cavitations in its wake as equally archaic.

In modern dentistry, there have been a few brilliant, maverick dentists who brought insight to the profession after suffering through the mercurial madness of mainstream dentistry to shed light and wisdom upon the mouth's mirror to health. Among these wise men is Dr. Weston Price, an early president of the American Dental Association who studied the link between nutrition and teeth in cultures around the world. Price was a pioneer in understanding how lethal bacterial build-up gets trapped in a root canal.

Maverick dentist Melvin Page contributed to the knowledge of the endocrine system, hormones, and oral health. He also calculated the perfect calcium to phosphorus ratio of 10:4 for bones and teeth, and the correct blood sugar level of 85 for optimal oral health. Page is the author of several books, including *Body Chemistry in Health & Disease* and *Degeneration-Regeneration*. He also created an anthropometrics system to bring the body chemistry back into balance.

Another dental pioneer, Dr. George Meinig, founder of the American Association of Endodontists (specialists in root canals procedures), who, after reading Dr. Weston Prices' 1174 detailed pages on root canal research, was inspired to write *Root Canal Cover-Up*. Meinig concluded that a "high percentage of chronic degenerative diseases can originate from root-filled teeth. The most frequent were heart and circulatory disease. The next most common diseases were those of the joints: arthritis and rheumatism." Meining also describes the healthy fluids that feed the teeth, "Undamaged dentin tubules contain a nutrient-dense fluid that keeps the teeth alive and healthy. These nutrients are supplied daily to each tubule by the artery that accompanies the nerve and vein in the root canal. The artery does this in the same way that other arteries supply nutrients to every cell of the body."

Renegade Robert O. Nara, DDS, who wrote *Money by the Mouthful,* writes about the dental industry's excessive "drill, fill, and bill" method of dentistry. He also studied the anti-bacterial and mouth rejuvenating aspects of salt and its use in oral care. He informs his readers that cavities are infections that can heal, and stated, "Literally millions of root canals have been done, when in reality there was no need for them in the first place...in my opinion the whole thing boils down to one simple fact: the dental establishment is scared to death that the public is going to realize that the entire profession has been making a living by repairing the results of a disease they could have been curing all along!"

In 1996, I spoke at the *International Herb & Aromatherapy Conference* in Arizona, and was happy to meet a very dear man who was handing out unique pamphlets about the hazards of fluoride and glycerin in toothpaste, who advised me to try brushing the teeth with soap! Curious, I tried brushing with a tiny dash of soap from a bar of Castile soap and it worked really well. Later, this experience led to my development of "Neem Enamelizer," which combines herbs, essential oils, and bio-saponins to brush the teeth. This pioneer was Gerard Judd and he wrote *Good Teeth from Birth to Death.*

The brilliant Dr. Hal Huggins, DDS, MSc, has contributed greatly to our current knowledge of the mouth's connection to the body. Huggins has both a Dentistry degree and a Master's degree in Immunology. He is an expert in blood and cellular chemistry with 40 years of research in Holistic Dentistry, and he has an abundant knowledge of minerals and teeth, organ function, mercury toxicity, and bacteria in jaw cavitations. Huggins developed protocols for removing mercury fillings, removing root canals, and cleaning up jaw cavitations. His institute, Huggins Applied Healing, is an excellent resource with a knowledgeable staff; they will answer any and all dental questions over the phone. (You can find their contact info in the resource section at the back of this book.) Hal authored *Uninformed Consent*, *It's All in Your Head*, *Why Raise Ugly Children* and *Mercury in My Molars*.

I take this opportunity to thank all of the dentists who have pioneered the idea of mercury-free practices and made the connection between our environment, a healthy mouth, and a healthy body.

Fillings: Heavy Metals by the Mouthful

Your parents may have warned you about handling the thermometer very carefully when you were a child for fear of breaking it. There was a good reason for this: thermometers contain mercury, which is the most toxic substance on earth, after plutonium. Today, if you break a compact florescent "environmental" light bulb (which contains mercury), it is just like breaking a thermometer. There are very strict Environmental Protection Agency (EPA) guidelines for its safe clean up.[5] Some of these caulions include:

---

[5] http://www.epa.gov/mercury/spills/

- Never use a vacuum cleaner to clean up mercury. The vacuum will put mercury into the air and increase exposure.

- Never use a broom to clean up mercury. It will break the mercury into smaller droplets and spread them.

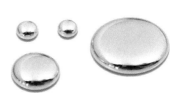

- Never pour mercury down a drain. It may lodge in the plumbing and cause future problems during plumbing repairs. If discharged, it can cause pollution of the septic tank or sewage treatment plant.

- Clothing that has come into direct contact with mercury should be *discarded*. Have all people and pets leave the room.

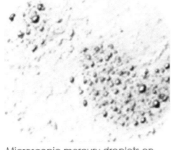

Microscopic mercury droplets on surface of a normal amalgam filling.

This should give you a good idea of how dangerous mercury is. Yet, somehow, someone saw fit to insert mercury in millions of mouths, implanted inches from our brains and the nasal, throat, and lung passageways! Dr. Boyd Haley[6] informs us that when mercury fillings are removed from the mouth (and

---

[6] Dr. Boyd Haley is a professor and chair of the chemistry department at the University of Kentucky. He has investigated the effect of mercury on tissues and on the mercury's biochemical effect in Alzheimer's disease and autism.

there is no change in substance to the filling once removed), this amalgam is considered toxic waste by the EPA and must be handled with a certain protocol to protect dental office personnel from mercury poisoning.

Dr. Haley reports, "Mercury is one of the most potent chemical inhibitors of thiol-sensitve enzymes, and mercury vapor easily penetrates in to the central nervous system. Amalgams leak mercury, this is a fact that any chemistry department can confirm[7]." Yet there are many dentists in a fog of mercury who will not heed this research.

The biggest exposure one will have to mercury in their lifetime is from fillings. The vapors from mercury fillings fume in the mouth 24 hours a day, 7 days a week, with more powerful bursts in response to chewing, teeth grinding, and drinking hot fluids. Chewing is the biggest culprit; if you chew gum, the vapor increases by 15,000%, causing galvanic currents (electric currents between the teeth). Mercury mixes with food being chewed,

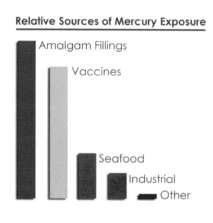

Relative Sources of Mercury Exposure

Amalgam Fillings

Vaccines

Seafood

Industrial

Other

---

[7] Haley, Boyd. "Dangers of Mercury based Amalgam Dental Fillings". Presented to: The Committee on Governmental Reform: Dental Amalgam Hearing November 14, 2002

and it disrupts the friendly bacteria of the gastro-intestinal tract. If you do not have a healthy diet, the resistance of the gum tissue decreases, and bacteria, fungus, and candida[8] thrive on mercury. Mercury also deeply affects the entire endocrine system. The glands of the endocrine system are an internal pharmacopeia of enzymes, hormones, and intricate chemical communication for the entire body, including insulin, testosterone, estrogen, and the thyroid, pituitary, and adrenalin glands. Mercury can slide into the binding receptor sites for the hormones, altering the original purpose of the hormones is altered.

Hal Huggins explains that when mercury reaches its destination tissue, it binds *tenaciously* and has many ways to express toxicity, including the alteration of cell membrane permeability, nerve impulses, enzyme and digestive function, genetic code, DNA repair, immune, protein synthesis, mitochondria energy production, and endocrine function.

But wait. There's more. *Much more.*

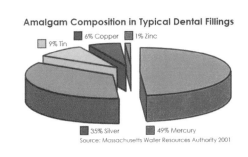

Amalgam Composition in Typical Dental Fillings

6% Copper 1% Zinc
9% Tin
35% Silver 49% Mercury
Source: Massachusetts Water Resources Authority 2001

The health hazards of mercury for dentists and patients have been debated since mercury was first introduced in

---

[8] Candida is challenging to clear up while mercury fillings are in the mouth; candida acts as a "protective" response to the mercury.

the 1830s. Mercury poisoning is *cumulative*. Muscle tremors are one of the first signs, and a whole host of adverse affects range from memory loss, gingivitis and receding gums, to chronic fatigue, multiple sclerosis, Parkinson's, and Alzheimer's. Many dental offices are in a fog of mercury and have "ambient mercury levels above Occupational Health and Safety regulations. Blood and urine samples of dentists found that 50 to 70% of those tested had above-normal levels of mercury. Inhalation of mercury vapors is the dentist's primary source of poisoning."[9]

Even though dentists fill teeth with mercury every day, in 1976, the *Journal of the American Dental Association* stated "No longer can the dental profession ignore the problem of mercury contamination in the dental office."[10]

A silver amalgam filling is created from a mixture of heavy metals. The amalgam used in silver-colored dental fillings contains approximately 49% metallic mercury, 35% silver, 9% tin, 6% copper, and trace amounts of zinc. When the amalgam is first mixed, it is a soft paste which is inserted into the tooth surface and hardens within 30 minutes. There are other filling options, although they also contain heavy metals, including gold crowns (with palladium, platinum, nickel and copper) and plastic fillings, also known as white fillings (often containing BPA and made with aluminum). Porcelain crowns, (expensive and

---

[9] *The Excruciating History of Dentistry*, Wynbrant 1998: 181

[10] *Journal of the American Dental Association*, Vol 92, Issue 6, 1195-1198, Copyright © 1976 by American Dental Association, LD Pagnotto and EM Comproni

not pure porcelain) which are backed onto a nickel thimble that covers the tooth, may also contain nickel and aluminum oxide. Nickel is a carcinogen that challenges the immune system when it is released from the filling. Composite fillings can also contain acrylate, aluminum, formaldehyde, hexane, hydroquinone, phenol, polyurethane, silane, strontium, toluene, and xylene. Braces and metal implants are also made with nickel. Metal titanium implants leak aluminum. This toxic list goes on and on, including other harmful materials used in the mouth to bond the fillings made with calcium hydroxide, containing toluene and potentially causing eczema and allergic reactions.

The best option, which is well tolerated by the body for a filling or restoration, is ceramics and ceramic-resin hybrids (different than porcelain) with special low temperature fusing. These ceramic options are generally bio-compatible and are strong enough for long term use. For more information about the brands and types of bonding options, see *Making the Right Dental Choices* by Dr. Bob Marshall in the resource section. Another option for cavity-infections that are very deep is the application of a composite resin, which avoids the drilling and filling process.

A Safe Harbour for Bacteria: Root Canals and Jaw Cavitations

> *"The mouth, the oral cavity literally is the basis of 70 to 90% of all medical problems. If you have a root canalled tooth you have a dead organ basically embalmed in the body"*
>
> *Dr. Gerald Smith*

A root-canalled tooth involves the removal of the complete internal structure of the tooth, including the nerve tissue, blood vessels, and cells. When a root canal is executed, it is impossible to clean the *three miles* of dentin tubules that compromise the dentin of a tooth that can get full of bacteria. (A root canal becomes a breeding ground for anaerobic bacteria and the release of *thiol-ethers* from the dead tissue in the mouth.) At this time, there appears to be no 100% effective method for cleaning these tiny tubules, so bacteria goes to the ligament that holds the tooth in place, which creates lethal bacteria that are squirted into the bloodstream every time you chew.

This leads us to the next fun subject: jaw cavitations. One of the hidden side-effects of modern dental procedures, and one which often produces no visible symptoms, are bacteria in the jawbone. A jaw cavitation (which is bacteria in the jaw) can lead to phantom tooth pain, neuralgia, and face pain. A jaw cavitation can have several causes, including: bacteria from an abscessed tooth, bacteria from an extracted tooth (wisdom tooth) site, or bacteria beneath a root canal or under an old crown. Jaw cavitations which are also known as *osteonecrotic lesions*, are infected necrotic bone, or, in simpler terms, a place where bacteria are beginning to eat away at the jawbone. As there are three miles of microscopic canals in each tooth, it is an excellent environment for bacteria to harbour. Even more dangerous than bacteria in the cavitation is the waste product of the bacteria, which is a neuro-toxin with a toxicity level that is off the charts. Jaw cavitations are not visible on x-rays, CAT scans, or through MRIs. Only a biological dentist can check by making a small incision and seeing if there is a "mushy" pocket in the bone. To clear up the cavitation, the site needs to be opened and the decay needs to be scraped off the bone[11] with the bacteria thoroughly removed and the site treated with ozone.

Think of it this way: cavities are in the teeth, and *cavitations* are in the jaw.

Fillings, extractions, root canals and cavitations are serious subjects that should only be consented to after thoughtful and well-informed consideration. All of these procedures require a highly-skilled biological dentist who has been thoroughly trained in the services of mercury filling removal, bio-compatible dentistry, and proper extraction methods above and beyond what was taught in dentistry school. Some holistic dentists only offer carrot juice and a tube of Crest while their office is still using outdated dental materials and methods.

To help you make an informed decision, ask your dentist the following questions before agreeing to any procedure:

Questions to Ask a Prospective Dentist

* Do they use bacteria water filters? The water used to rinse your mouth may be laden with

---

[11] Many biological dentists follow the "Huggins three mile limit", which requires a patient to rest for one hour after the procedure so that a blood clot forms and healing takes place.

harmful bacteria. The bacterium stagnates in the waterlines!

- Do they do Biocompatible Testing on a patient-by-patient basis to check compatibility with dental materials? The dentist can test your blood to find out what dental materials your body can accept. About 60% of dental materials will suppress your immune system.

- Do they use ozone and/or lasers for cleaning areas of the mouth and newly filled teeth?

- Does the dentist use a laser to bond a new inlay or crown? Laser bonding is strong and avoids toxic dental cements.

- Do they use phase contrast microscopes? This procedure is where they take bacteria from the gum line to determine the health of the gums in advance, long before periodontal disease sets in.

- Is it a mercury-free dental practice?

- Do they have a full protocol for removing amalgam fillings? This would include dental dams, oxygen supplied to patient, vitamin C, and an air filtration system placed near the mouth to suck up mercury vapors.

- Do they have intravenous Vitamin C drips available during procedures?

- Do you they use digital x-rays? These have 90% less radiation.

- Do they use intra-oral cameras? These transmit an image to a screen so that you and the dentist can look at your mouth together.

- Does the dentist use a brand-new *drill bur* for dental restorations?

- Is the dentist properly trained (more than a weekend course) in the removal of mercury?

Preparing for a Dental Appointment

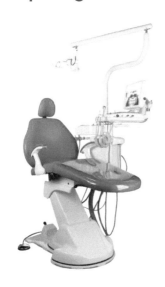

Even if you are giving your teeth a whole new daily clean, if they teeth have been neglected for a while or you have had previous dental work that is no longer desired (like a mercury filling), you will need to visit that wonderful new biological dentist you have found.

Professional dental cleanings will reduce tartar deposits on the teeth, but cannot stop the re-growth of acid-loving bacteria, nor will a cleaning strengthen or protect teeth. After a deep scaling by a hygienist, oral bacteria are dislodged and bacterium goes into the blood stream, challenging your immune system. The body responds to this perceived attack by releasing white blood cells to combat the invading microbes and the resulting inflammation. After a cleaning, many harmful bacteria are present in the saliva and will reestablish themselves on the teeth and in the blood stream. In fact, one is not allowed to donate blood for 48 hours after a dental cleaning.

Prepare for your appointment at least three weeks in advance by doing the following:

- Proceed with the 8 Steps of Successful Self-Dentistry (see Chapter 6).

- Build your immune system with vitamin C, 1000 to 2000 mg per day depending on your health and bowel tolerance. Lipospheric has the best absorbability, and taking 5/1000mg packets is the closest thing to taking vitamin C intravenously. If you are going to the dentist for more serious work than a cleaning, be advised that taking vitamin C orally reduces the numbing effect of Novocain and anesthetic.

- Check saliva and urine pH with litmus paper, and maintain alkaline levels.

- Bring your own spring water with salt added for rinsing.

- Anoint gums with Healthy Gum Drops or Yogi Tooth Serum before, during, and after the visit, and ask the hygienist to floss your teeth with one of these serums.

- A great tip from Hal Huggins for very inflamed gums: thoroughly and vigorously swish mouth with salt water every hour for 2 days (half a teaspoon of pure sodium chloride to a glass of warm water), and on the half hour rinse with *sodium ascorbate* vitamin C powder. Note: this is *not* the acid form of vitamin C (ascorbate acid), which is acidic and only has a pH of one. Huggins explains that salt kills the bacteria and vitamin C creates electrons (unhealthy tissue is saturated with protons and healthy tissue is saturated with electrons).

• After the dentist – extra vitamin C

Even if you are only doing the minimal oral hygienic work that is required (i.e. regular cleanings), you are really just getting your teeth scraped with tools. And this brings us back to our core focus... keeping the enamel healthy. It is true that there's probably no better way to remove old, overgrown calculus than to have a hygienist completely scrape it off, yet if you practice proper gum care, maintain 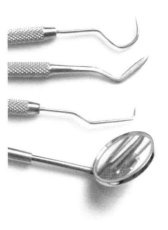 awareness of proper alkalinity, brush properly, and floss with Tooth Serums, over the course of a few weeks you are going to correct numerous issues that will inhibit the calculus from building-up.

4. Processed Food Equals Processed Teeth

The mouth is part of the body, and its health and vitality are directly linked to the nutrition provided by each meal we ingest. Our teeth are taken care of externally by brushing and flossing, however, *internally* we feed the health of our teeth through the food and water we absorb.

In our industrialized era, processed food is standard fare. For many people it is quite common to eat frozen dinners, sugary snacks, preservatives, additives, dyes, soda pop, and fluffy white bread. 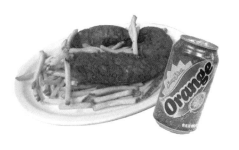 Thankfully, there has been resurgence toward eating whole unprocessed foods, pastured foods, wild foods, and super-foods. In this next section we will explore how certain foods can cause or cure a cavity.

Decay of the tooth enamel is less about the food that gets stuck between it and more about the nutrients that get sucked *into* it. Dental decay occurs in two different ways: internally and externally. External factors can include food in the mouth, acidity, strength of the gum tissue, teeth grinding, and bacteria. External factors play a role, yet they are not the *initiating* factors in oral decay. Teeth are alive. Much of what they are made of can *regenerate*, and this is why internal factors that nourish the teeth are so important. Real foods, hormonal balance, minerals, and fluid exchange in and out of the teeth are key. When the teeth are healthy, they are like trees, drawing their nourishment from the roots and the blood and digestive system are the soil. Nourishing fluid moves from the pulp chamber through to the dentin and out to the enamel. Stress, processed food, and inadequate nutrition will reverse this precious flow, and bacteria and acids from the mouth will be drawn into the tooth.

The tooth is full of pores, and the pores in a healthy tooth have a blood supply that washes them clean from the inside out. Brushing keeps the plaque away and the gum tissue in good health, yet the tooth is cleansed *internally*. The serum of the blood actually pushes through the tooth and out into the mouth. Beyond the digestive processes and absorption of vitamins and minerals, the hypothalamus (the master switch for the endocrine/glandular system) releases a hormone, which in turn stimulates the parotid (a salivary gland) to release its parotid hormone. When the parotid hormone is balanced, the fluid travels from the pulp chamber through the dentin, then through the enamel and into the mouth. It is a lovely, perfect process.

Refined sugar, processed food, additives, preservatives, stress (high cortisol levels), mercury, and fluoride reverse the fluid flow of the teeth, and fluid flow is vital to oral health. This movement of fluid is similar to the movement of fluid between cells. In a conversation between Dr. Hal Huggins and one of his mentors, Dr. Ralph Steinman, Dr. Steinman explains:

> "By altering the function of the endocrine glands, that fluid flow could be reversed, such that the tooth sucks in bacteria, acids and other things from the mouth into the tooth. Can the fluid flow be restored to a mouth that is experiencing decay and acidic saliva? Yes, simply by changing the diet. Most of the "flow-in" foods are refined food... About the age of two or three years, the permanent teeth are forming within the jawbone. If there is deficiency of vitamin C, D or A during calcification [when the teeth are forming], a tooth less resistant to decay will be produced."[12]

Furthermore, the thyroid is an important gland which can influence oral ecology. The thyroid, as part of the endocrine system, also influences the nourishing fluid flow from the roots to the pulp chamber through the dentin to the enamel. Low thyroid function can reverse the flow, bringing bacteria into the bloodstream.

Drs. Edward and May Mellanby, who discoverered that vitamin D[13] was the cause of rickets, also did research on the nutritional factors affecting tooth

---

[12] Huggins, *Why Raise Ugly Kids?* 1981: 145-146

[13] Vitamin D is a steroidal precursor hormone that is lavishly supplied to our bodies by the sun's interaction with our skin, plays an

formation (occlusion). Their research confirmed that when enamel and dentine are injured by attrition of dental caries, the teeth are alive and respond to the infection by sending odontoblasts into the dental pulp where the damaged tissue is, laying down what is called *secondary dentin.* In 1922, May Mellanby's further studies showed that a diet high in Vitamin D, phosphorus, and

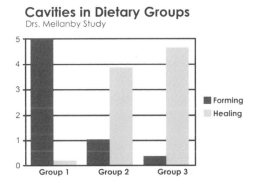

Cavities in Dietary Groups
Drs. Mellanby Study

calcium-forming minerals (silica and magnesium), formed a solid, thick foundation of secondary dentine, whether the original structure of the tooth was good or bad. However, if the diet was rich in processed cereals, grains, and lacking in vitamin D and minerals, the secondary dentine was calcified (formed) more poorly. This brings up the finer points of diet that go beyond whole foods and includes foods that are mineral rich, foods high in fat of the soluble vitamins E, D3, A and K2, and how well foods are being absorbed. For proper absorption of nutrients, the body needs healthy intestinal function, ample digestive enzymes, and hydrochloric acid. The following must also be eliminated for digestive health: anti-nutrients, foods that block mineral absorption, phytic acid, and foods that have no minerals (like processed food).

Processed Food Equals Processed Teeth

In another study, the Mellanbys divided 62 children into three different diet groups.[14] Group One ate their normal diet plus oatmeal (rich in phytic acid). Group Two ate their normal diet plus vitamin D, and Group Three ate a grain-free diet and took vitamin D (this group was grain free, but not sugar or carbohydrate free). In Group One, the rickets producing-effect of the oatmeal's phytic acid inhibited healing and encouraged new cavities.[15] In Group Two, most cavities healed and fewer new ones formed. In the Third Group, nearly all cavities healed and very few new cavities developed.

Further to these discoveries, Dr. Weston Price also had success curing tooth decay by feeding underprivileged children one nutritious meal a day.[16] The children had meals with fresh cod liver oil[17] (high in vitamin D) and fresh alkaline broths. The diet was not grain free; however, the bread used was sour dough (fermented) and made from freshly stone-milled grain, which reduces the phytic acid tremendously. The children also ate a high-vitamin unpasteurized (raw) butter, which was made from summer grass-fed cows. This kind of butter is one of the richest sources of vitamin K2. These vital fat soluble vitamins give the body instructions to remineralize bones. Today, we also know that vitamin D3 and K2 are completely synergistic and more important than calcium for forming bones.

---

[14] The *British Medical Journal* 1932, 1:507.
[15] Mellanby, *Journal of Physiology* 1949 109: 488-533
[16] Price, *Nutrition and Physical Degeneration* : 290
[17] Effective re-mineralization, Dr. Price found a 40% increase in healing cavities with cod liver oil.

Phytates in food are found among grains, beans, seeds, and nuts. Phytic acid, known as an anti-nutrient, tightly binds phosphorus and blocks its bioavailability. Phytic acid can also chelate and block other important minerals such as zinc, calcium, and iron, from the body and can inhibit enzymes that are needed to digest food. Thus, our ancestors in various indigenous cultures had many recipes that stone-ground, soaked and *fermented* grains, nuts, beans, and seeds. Stone grinding and fermenting foods is a lost art, and currently grains and cereals are often rancid and processed with bromine. Commercially-grown foods, using synthetic phosphate fertilizers, contain higher amounts of phytic acid. Whole grains have more phytic acid than processed grains. If each meal of your daily diet revolves around grains, like oatmeal or cereal for breakfast, and rice for dinner, or if you are eating meat, eggs, and dairy that are grain-fed, you may need to reconsider what is nourishing your family[18]. A cavity-free mouth has a pH of 7 corresponding to a healthier oral and body/gut ecology, and is further benefited by the availability and assimilation of fat soluble vitamins and minerals in the blood stream, which can be used by the body to re-mineralize the teeth.

Melvin Page, DDS, author of many books, including *Your Body Is Your Best Doctor*,[19] discovered that

---

[18] Wheat and grains contain lectins, anti-nutrients, which interfere with digestive/absorptive activities and can shift the balance in bacterial flora shown to cause problems with normal gut metabolism. When grains are consumed through animal foods omega 6/omega 3 ratios are imbalanced.

[19] 2001, Authors Choice Press

tooth decay can be kept at bay when the calcium phosphorus ratio in the blood is 10:4 and blood sugar is at a healthy 85. *Why is this?*

When blood sugar levels are too high it creates insulin resistance, which creates a state of inflammation in the body. Maintaining low daily glucose levels is a good way to have a positive impact on the health of our teeth and gums.

Phosphorous levels in the blood should be maintained at a level above 3.5. If the phosphorus serum is above 3.5, the fluid flows in a normal, healthy direction: up into the roots, nourishing the teeth like tree roots. This fluid flow creates nourishment and inner self-cleansing of all the tiny tubules. If, however, the level of phosphorous serum drops below 3.5 the fluid flow reverses going from the mouth to the tooth and into the bloodstream, resulting in decay. Dr. Melvin Page ran more than two thousand blood chemistry tests and discovered that no cavities occurred when the calcium to phosphorus ratio was in a proportion of 10 to 4 in the blood. Forty-two years later, the Department of Dental Research of the United States Air Force confirmed Dr. Page's findings of a calcium phosphorus ratio to be correct. Dr. Page also discerned from these tests that the blood sugar level should be approximately 85. "Thus, the basic research of Dr. Page uncovered the knowledge that white sugar and refined carbohydrates increases serum calcium. Calcium is drawn from the bone tissue and is then carried in the serum calcium."[20]

---

[20] International Foundation for Nutrition & Health http://www.ifnh.org/Bio%20Page%20.htm

With prolonged spikes in blood sugar, minerals, including calcium, are leeched from the bones, and the body begins to de-mineralize.

This is tooth care that goes far beyond mere brushing of the teeth.

Key Nutritional Guidelines Learned from These studies:

- All grains, beans, and nuts must be soaked and fermented to remove and evolve phytic acid.
- Eat fresh, whole foods.
- Eat *zero* processed foods.
- Eat fruits and vegetables that are organic and grown in mineral-rich soils.
- Eat herbs that are mineral-rich and made into smoothies and teas, like horsetail and nettles.
- Get sufficient sunlight or take Vitamin D3 supplements.
- Eat grass fed unpasteurized ghee, butter, or K2 supplements.
- Animal foods are best wild or organic and **100%** grass-fed "pastured:" organic dairy is best raw.

You may be surprised to learn that tooth decay is not exclusively about sugar. In fact, if you put sugar on bacteria in a Petri dish the bacteria *will not* eat the sugar because it does not *like* sugar. Decay is not caused by sugar touching the teeth, but by sugar *in the diet*, which causes depletion in nutrition that can result in tooth decay. Sugar creates acidity in the mouth and intestinal tract, which is the opposite of what healthy saliva needs. It also leeches minerals from the teeth, bringing phosphorus and calcium levels into imbalance, which is a formula for decay.

Refined sugar is also disruptive to the endocrine system, the hypothalamus, the adrenal glands, the pituitary glands, the pineal glands, and the hormonal secretions of cortisol, progesterone, DHEA, testosterone, and estrogen. In one well-known study[21], rats were given sugary soda to drink. It did not cause decay on the tooth, yet, in another part of the study, when they injected the rat's stomachs with soda, the cavities started forming!

Some of the best research on the relationship between processed food and dental health comes from Dr. Weston Price.[22] In the 1920s, he was president of the *American Dental Association*, and he travelled to many cultures that were still eating their ancestral diets. (At the time this basically referred to cultures that hadn't yet been colonized by Europeans and had not been exposed to white bread, white sugar and chemicals.) These people were eating the traditional diets that their ancestors had been eating for centuries. Dr. Weston studied their facial structure, jaws, and teeth, as well as the jaws of skeletons found in the area. What he found was that prior to the 19th century, there were very few cavities. He found approximately one cavity out of 1,000 skulls! This is a total reversal of today's statistics.

The bottom line? All processed food can lead to decay. The science is simple and can be summed

---

[21] Huggins, *Why Raise Ugly kids*, 1981:147
[22] http://www.westonaprice.org

up in one sentence: processed and refined foods can disrupt the digestion and the endocrine system, altering the flow of nutrients to the teeth. It is less than ideal for your teeth and gums when the internal environment has collapsed, the nutrition is absent, and there are a few generations of ancestors with depleted nutrition in your genealogy.

Teeth are created to be fed from the *inside* in order to nourish the dentin and the saliva. So, here is the best formula: no processed food, no white sugar, no white flour, no soda, no saccharine, no high fructose corn syrup, and absolutely zero convenience store foods -- *zero!* Well, none that is, if you want to be healthy.

5. Oral Care for Children

We all remember learning about the tooth fairy. Yet, how many of us ever learned about actual *teeth* when we were kids? Even though we are all grown up now, it is never too late to learn, and it is actually a perfect time to teach our children about dental health. When our children are young, we have a fresh opportunity to share ideas about the body's ability to regenerate and implement ideal dietary and oral care practices.

Sometimes helping children brush their teeth, or getting children to brush their own teeth, can feel a lot like herding cats! Even though you may try to bribe, convince, or break out in song and dance, cheerfully chanting, *"If you get up in the morning... and you want to find something to do, brush your teeth ch ch ch ch, ch ch ch ch"*,[23] and your child *still* closes her mouth against the toothbrush, you should know, though your dentist may not say so, that brushing *is not* everything. Even when children do brush their teeth, or teenagers for that matter, are they doing a thorough job? Is their brushing completely effective in clearing away all the plaque?

It all begins before we are born. Generally, newborns are born without teeth, yet their teeth are already forming. In fact, a baby's teeth have been forming all along in-utero, so certainly pre-conception and

---

[23] "Brush Your Teeth" by Songwriters: Raffi Cavoukian and Louise Cullen

pre-natal nutrition are key, especially ensuring that the fat-soluble vitamins such as A, D3, and K2, are part of one's daily nutrition. Breastfeeding is also of prime importance to taking care of your baby's teeth. There is a lot of research being done that shows bottle-fed babies end up with rotting front teeth, which is caused by the lack of nutrients in the formula and sometimes because the formula's bacteria stay on the teeth while the baby is sleeping.

With a new baby, you have a golden opportunity to celebrate a healthy, balanced human being, and a good place to start is with purity in diet. If you never introduce your child to highly processed foods and junk food, the odds are excellent that he or she will not develop a craving for them. My recommendation is to offer no processed foods whatsoever, including formula and processed juices - even apple juice from the health-food store. The best thing for your baby to drink is pure spring water and breast milk. Certain herbal teas, sipped at room temperature, like chamomile and nettle, are also a lovely option.

As the child grows and starts eating more solid foods, you will need to include plenty of fat-soluble vitamins and mineral rich food. As the teeth begin to come in, even though it is too early to brush, you can still take care of them by wiping each tooth with a cloth, just to make sure that it is clear of any food or acidic buildup.

There is an informative book about children's teeth, called *Why Raise Ugly Kids?* by Dr. Hal Huggins. In it, he explains orthodontics and methods of creating space in the mouth for teeth to come in and move around properly, pointing out that poor diet is a major cause of the jaw developing abnormally. This is particularly true for the pre-natal diet. Nutrition is a significant factor that influences the development of the entire mouth, not just the teeth, and should include a healthy pre-natal diet, breast feeding and raising children on real, unprocessed foods. If this were the norm, wisdom teeth extractions and orthodontists would be scarce. Dentist Dr. Strauss, who specializes in sleep apnea, further validates this thinking by explaining that when the palate is broad there is more room for teeth and breathing. He explains, "When you look at the percentage of people in civilized societies seeing orthodontists, and then when you add to it the lack of breastfeeding, which generally is a positive way of expanding the size of the palate, moving the jaw further forward and having a larger mouth to hold the teeth, it's not surprising that so many *have* sleep apnea in civilized society.[24]"

Children are young, vital, and, of course growing, so childhood cavities are not a degenerative, aging issue. There is a common misconception that it is normal for kids to have cavities. However, the truth is that cavities can absolutely be avoided. Early childhood dental filling and drilling does not stop tooth decay: it only plugs the problem rather than getting to the root of the issue. This is because the symptom is being removed while the real issue -- the cause of the decay – is not being addressed.

[24] http://articles.mercola.com/sites/articles/archive/2011/05/21/dr-arthur-strauss-on-sleep-apnea.aspx

Tooth decay in babies and toddlers is *never* caused by breastfeeding[25]. Children grow rapidly in their sleep, and nighttime nursing, which has been done since the beginning of time, has never caused a cavity. Mothers who are breastfeeding, take care! You must get tons of nutrient-dense food and fresh water to nourish yourself and your child.

If a brown lesion appears on your child's tooth, keep it clean with salt rinses, baking soda, clay, and botanicals, while keeping your eye on it because it is still at a stage where the damage can be reversed. Do not make the mistake of thinking that a lesion means you are on a slope towards a cavity. It *could* be, yet a carie is positively reversible. When the brown lesion comes in, the dentin inside the tooth is sending out odontoblasts, which send new cellular growth to the area. The tooth *is* healing itself. The brown area, when healed, still has good, strong enamel.

In ancient times, cavities in children were a rare occurrence. Today, one of the biggest health concerns in North America and Europe affecting little ones more than any other age group is dental decay, or ECC (Early Childhood Caries). Beyond brushing, the internal factors that nourish the teeth are so important: real foods, hormonal balance, minerals, fat soluble vitamins, and a healthy fluid exchange through the teeth. Stress, processed foods, and inadequate nutrition negatively affect the fluid flow that nourishes teeth for children and

---

[25] For further reading: http://mothering.com/health/big-bad-cavities-breastfeeding-is-not-the-cause

teens. To prevent cavities, always provide whole foods, and examine what sources of vitamins and minerals your child is getting. Remember, some whole grains and nuts need traditional methods of soaking and fermenting to reduce the phytic acids.

Bonding agents (sealants) are often recommended by dentists to prevent cavities in children. This is done by etching the tooth and filing the micro-pores with a plastic resin, sealing the pits and fissures of the teeth, which are often sites for decay. This seems like a practical intervention, however, the sealants leak a plastic chemical called _Bisphenol A_ (toxic for adults _and_ children), and the sealants only last about a year. They may "protect" the teeth from bacteria, yet some bacteria are still trapped underneath, leaving the tooth even weaker when the sealant is gone. (The sealants are not removed, so where do they go?) A new technique has been developed to prevent trapping bacteria underneath by cleaning the tooth beforehand with a drill burr, which removes part of the tooth. When this is done, one is ultimately left with a tiny cavity filling on a new tooth to prevent a cavity filling. _Does this make sense?_

At about eighteen months, teach your children to swish with salt water and to start brushing their teeth. If the child's teeth are set close together, you will want to begin flossing them. (You can rest their head on your lap and floss their teeth.) Make it a fun family activity and take your time. This will create a foundation of great oral health for a lifetime.

Sharing the body's innate wisdom with your child creates a strong foundation of vitality. Most parents consider the college fund to be the most valuable gift that they may provide for their children's future.

Teeth are valuable, and endowing your child with a legacy of understanding that the body and the mouth are dynamic and regenerative will serve them throughout their thriving lives, far exceeding in long-term value the gift of a college education.

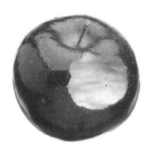

6. Successful Self-Dentistry in Eight Steps

"Freedom is the first step and the last."

Krishnamurti

This section explores eight simple steps of successful self-dentistry that you can integrate into your daily life. You may have been brushing your teeth the same way for 10, 20, 40, or 80 years, and it is now time to breathe freshness into your oral care routine! If you use these steps every day, you will be amazed at how effective

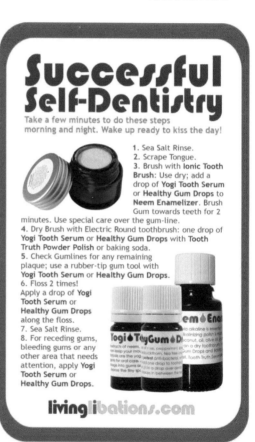

Successful Self-Dentistry

Take a few minutes to do these steps morning and night. Wake up ready to kiss the day!

1. Sea Salt Rinse.
2. Scrape Tongue.
3. Brush with **Ionic Tooth Brush**: Use dry; add a drop of **Yogi Tooth Serum** or **Healthy Gum Drops** to **Neem Enamelizer**. Brush Gum towards teeth for 2 minutes. Use special care over the gum-line.
4. Dry Brush with Electric Round toothbrush: one drop of **Yogi Tooth Serum** or **Healthy Gum Drops** with **Tooth Truth Powder Polish** or baking soda.
5. Check Gumlines for any remaining plaque; use a rubber-tip gum tool with **Yogi Tooth Serum** or **Healthy Gum Drops**.
6. Floss 2 times! Apply a drop of **Yogi Tooth Serum** or **Healthy Gum Drops** along the floss.
7. Sea Salt Rinse.
8. For receding gums, bleeding gums or any other area that needs attention, apply **Yogi Tooth Serum** or **Healthy Gum Drops**.

livinglibations.com

they are at preventing decay, the onset of colds,

acidic saliva, plaque build-up, gum bleeding, inflammation, and more.

Ideally, these steps are completed morning and night, because within six hours of brushing your teeth, plaque starts to return. After 2-4 days of neglect, gum tissue sends warnings to your immune system that something is up, and the immune system responds by sending white blood cells to help out. This causes a breakdown of the collagen fibers which hold teeth to the jaw bone. Within a week or two of neglect, biofilm forms bacterial colonies. This is when gums may start to bleed, especially when flossing.

We often fear the unknown, so get to *know* your mouth. Get a dental mirror with a light, or an intra-oral camera from EBay, and get acquainted with those back molars. This Successful Self-Dentistry protocol will keep your mouth, teeth, gums, and saliva in pristine condition, so that every day feels like you've been to the dental hygienist for a cleaning.

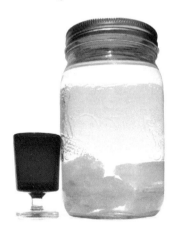

Step One: The Salt Rinse

Most people have salt in their homes, so you can start with this effective step right away. Salt eliminates microbes and makes the mouth alkaline, creating a neutral palate for brushing. It can come in handy after a meal when it is less-than-ideal to brush your teeth. This is especially important after you have eaten citrus or grapefruit, to neutralize the acids right away.

Begin by getting a mason jar and a shot glass for each member of your family; mix 1 oz of salt to 16oz of hot, almost boiled, spring water (or non fluoridated, non-chlorinated water). The hot water activates and dissolves the salt into brine. A drop of *Healthy Gum Drops* or *Yogi Tooth Serum* may be added and shaken (not stirred) into your brine. To start the routine, pour yourself a small shot glass of the salt mixture: swish, swish, swish, and spit.

Step Two: Scraping the Tongue

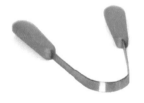

The coating of the tongue is home to many microbes and mucus that migrate from the alimentary canal. You can buy a tongue scraper at any health food store, or you can use the back of a spoon. Simply scrape your tongue from back to front, and you will see the plaque being removed. Rinse the scraper in hot water, and scrape again until your tongue is clear, usually in 2-3 scrapes. Tip: add one of the tooth serums to the scraper. Scraping the tongue helps to eliminate morning breath. And you will find that with improved nutrition, there will be less to scrape.

Step Three: Brushing the Gums

Brushing the gums the right way is important, so pay special attention to brushing the gums *toward* the teeth and use special care over the gum line (the union of teeth and gums). Brush as gently as you can, and move your brush from the gums towards the teeth (downward on the top teeth and upward on the bottom teeth). Use a soft bristled, manual dry brush for this step, and combine a tiny drop of *Neem Enamelizer* (to optimally allow the process of re-mineralization) with a drop of *Yogi Tooth Serum* or *Healthy Gum Drops*.

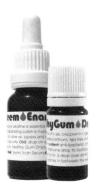

Take a moment to be mindful about this step. Sit down on the toilet seat or on the edge of the bathtub and relax! You can even go outside, or brush with a friend. Make it fun! The old days of standing over the sink with the water running and spitting out mouthfuls of foaming sodium laurel sulfate are over!

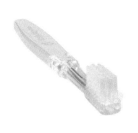

By the way, my favorite manual toothbrush is the light-activated ionic tooth brush. This brush creates negative ions in your saliva that draw away 40% of the plaque automatically. It is simple – just by ionizing and alkalinizing the saliva in the mouth the amount of plaque reduction is incredible.

Step Four: Polishing the Teeth

This step creates smooth, slippery teeth that you will enjoy gliding your tongue over. This assures that any leftover plaque is removed and can create whiter, brighter teeth. For this step, use a round-head electric brush. I have tried a wide variety of electric brushes on the market and find that a simple rechargeable brush ($25) does the job very well. The small round-headed electric brush is effective because it easily enters areas that are not effectively reached by a manual brush. Add one drop of *Yogi Tooth Serum* or *Healthy Gum Drops* and a dash of *Tooth Truth Polish* or a homemade combination of salt and baking soda. With a little energy, the sticky plaque and biofilm will be removed in one to two minutes.

For this brushing stage you are focusing on the teeth (avoiding the gums) and getting them smooth and shiny.

Step Five: Checking the Gum Lines

Now for step five: check the inner and outer gum lines with your tongue. You will often find that there is plaque right at the gum line (aka the sulca). For this area, there are rubber-tipped gum tools and/or sulca brushes. Apply a drop of serum to the tool and go over the gum line. This step is very important, as the health of the gums is directly related to the health of the teeth. The gums hold the teeth in place and allow them to stay strong. The gums also cover thousands of tiny filaments that attach the tooth to the jaw, so taking good care of this area will prevent plaque from building up. Go over the gum line of each tooth, both on the inside and on the outside.

Step Six: Flossing

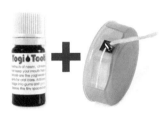

Now you are ready to floss. If you are a person who dislikes flossing, you are in for a pleasant surprise, because when you floss with one of the Tooth Serums it is fun and refreshing! Plus, if you already like flossing, you are going to enjoy it even more. Cardiologist Dr. Stephen Sinatra, states that flossing one's teeth daily can add seven years to a person's life!

To floss, take off a long strand. Put a drop of Yogi Tooth Serum or Healthy Gum Drops on your index finger and run the floss between your thumb and index finger to coat it with the serum. Wind the floss around the fingers and slide in between the teeth, up and down, and back and forth. Get clean in between, take care to pass the floss in the interstices and around the necks of the teeth where food and plaque buildup.

Step Seven: Final Rinse

Swish and rinse again. Do one more shot of your handy, dandy mouth-rinse brine: swish, swish, swish, and spit. The salt water and essential oils will coat your entire mouth, discouraging the growth of bacteria and nurturing the tissue. This swishing step could also be a time when you can alternate rinses among the brine, magnesium, and iodine (further details in **More Teeth Tips** section).

Step Eight: Extra Care

In our oral care kit we include a pocket oral irrigator called a *Vita Pik*. It is like a mini shower head that flushes out the gum line, irrigating places that flossing, brushing, and scraping cannot reach. 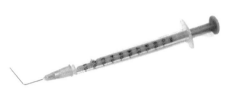 This mini irrigator is finer than a water-pick because it is made from a blunt-ended syringe and will rinse the microbes that previous steps may have missed.

Pour a small amount of your homemade mouthwash-brine with one drop of a Tooth Serum into your shot glass to fill the irrigator. Simply draw your mixture up into the syringe, flush the sulca and interstices of each tooth, and take extra care in areas that need special attention. This will dissolve remaining biofilm and microbes while revitalizing the gum tissue. Lastly, apply a drop of Tooth Serum to the gums to soothe tissue, fortify microbial protection, and freshen breath.

That is the protocol in eight simple steps. You can start right away with just salt and baking soda if you do not have the other items, yet. If you follow these steps daily – hopefully twice a day – you will notice a remarkable difference in your oral ecology.

Simple Review of the Eight Steps

1. Keep a salt water solution close to where you brush your teeth. Add a drop of Yogi Tooth Serum or Healthy Gum drops. Start with a salt water rinse before brushing.

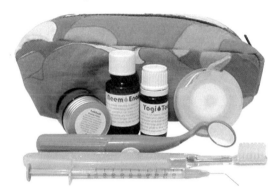

2. Scrape the tongue 2-3 times.

3. Brush the gums, paying special attention to brushing gums towards the teeth and using special care over the gum line. Use a soft, dry brush and apply a tiny drop of *Neem Enamelizer* with a drop of *Yogi Tooth Serum* or *Healthy Gum Drops*.

4. Polish the teeth with a dry, electric round-headed tooth brush. Add a drop of *Healthy Gum Drops* or Yogi *Tooth Serum* with a dash of baking soda, clay, or *Tooth Truth Powder Polish*.

5. Check the gum lines for any remaining plaque by using a rubber-tipped gum tool, sulca brush and/ or inter-proximal brush (like a tiny bottle brush for

in between the teeth) with a drop of *Yogi Tooth Serum* or *Healthy Gum Drops*.

6. Floss 2 times! Apply a drop of *Yogi Tooth Serum* or *Healthy Gum Drops* along the floss.

7. Use salt rinse – vigorous swish and spit.

8. Pay extra care to areas that need special attention, apply a drop of Serum and massage into gum line, sensitive areas, or use the *Vita Pik* to rinse gum pockets with salt water.

7. **The Benefits of Botanicals**

Essential oils address the circumstances that lead to a compromised immune system, including unwanted bacteria, viral loads, chronic inflammation, and a congested lymph system. The use of genuine essential oils originated as a medical therapy based on the pharmacological benefits of essential plant extracts. Since its origin, the modern commercialization and synthetic production of fragrances and flavors has relegated the aromatherapeutic use of essential oils to a frivolous realm of perfumery and potpourri.

These special plant extracts, which are different than herbal tinctures, homeopathics, or food supplements, are the distilled essences of the plants that bear their names. Each authentic essence is distilled slowly and at low temperatures. This captures the integrity of hundreds of botanical plant compounds and trace substances known as *secondary metabolites*.

Secondary metabolites are also known as *adaptogens* and are different from the DNA and primary structure of the plant. These adaptogenic substances are the plant hormones, phenols, and pheromones that attract pollinators, repel insects, and are part of the unique individual expression of the plant. The molecules in these substances mirror our human hormones, enzymes, and neuro-transmitters, representing the biological compatibility between humans and plant essences. Understandably, they can have a powerful effect on our health.

The Benefits of Botanicals

Essential oils and supercritical extracts are the key to our Living Libations formulas. They are highly concentrated, and with some of our botanicals, a whole plant is required to create only *one drop* of oil. The distinctive lipid-soluble structure of essential oils allow them to penetrate the lipid matrix and benefit the immune system, in addition to which the mosaic effect of the combined botanicals creates an effect of thousands of plant compounds. Some plant compounds will reduce inflammation, while others will have an antibacterial effect, and others an antiseptic one. Many essential oils combine all of these compounds.

Production of the formulas begins with good soil and organic growing practices, or sustainable wild-crafting of the plant matter. Each botanical ingredient is gathered at the right time of day to ensure the maximum amount of essence in the part of the plant being distilled. The right distillation method, a long, slow distillation, for example, further ensures that the maximum amount of compounds and trace elements are captured in every drop.

Our Living Libations formulas are anti-microbial, anti-fungal, anti-bacterial, and anti-inflammatory, and easily penetrate the lipid matrix of the gums. They send

nutrients to the blood vessels and molecules, and reach the dentine, nerves, and roots of the teeth. They get the circulation and the lymph system going. Elements such as *seabuckthorn berry* in the *Healthy Gum Drops* help to regenerate gum tissue.

The Benefits of Botanicals

Essential oils are also potent in oxygen radical absorption capacity, or ORAC[26], and have been found to be among some of the most powerful antioxidants. Clove and cinnamon are very high in ORAC capability, and have impressive properties for eliminating bacteria.

Essential oils have a dynamic interaction with the body, both physically and psychologically. Pure aromatic molecules offer a direct route through the blood-brain barrier into the centre of the mind, the hypothalamus. When the molecules reach the hypothalamus, the brain releases neurotransmitters, among them encephalin, endorphins, serotonin, and noradrenalin. Encephalin reduces pain and produces pleasant euphoric sensations and feelings of well being. Serotonin is relaxing and calming. Noradrenalin revitalizes the mind.

Certain essential oils can affect the autonomic nervous system, relax the heartbeat, deepen breathing, regulate the digestive process, and evoke inspiration. They can reach the limbic system in seconds, and once there the aromatic molecules continue their journey towards the lungs where they pass through the moist delicate walls of the alveoli and into the blood capillaries. From the capillaries, the tiny molecules flow to the heart, circulatory, and lymph systems and so access all organs and systems in the body.

Essential oils are extremely potent, often hundreds of times stronger than the herbal extraction of the same plant. Each oil has hundreds of botanical

[26] Oxygen Radical Absorbance Capacity

chemical components that work synergistically. Genuine distillations of plants, flowers, seeds, roots, and trees have been used medicinally for centuries.

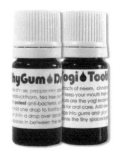

Healthy Gum Drops contains super-critical extracts and essences of seabuckthorn berry, rose otto, oregano, peppermint, clove, tea tree, cinnamon, and thyme linalool.

Yogi Tooth Serum is made with potent extracts of neem, cinnamon, clove, cayenne, mastic, and cardamom to provide oral care support. This combination of ancient Vedic botanicals, Yogi Tooth Serum, is the yogi secret of anti-bacterial, anti-viral, and anti-fungal oral care.

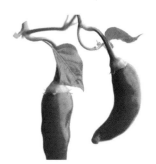

Cayenne, *Capsicum frutescens.* Ours is a super-critical extract with catalytic, antibacterial, antiseptic, and stimulating properties. The *capsaicin* compound in cayenne is also a topical vasodilator which stimulates blood circulation.

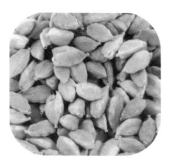

Cardamom, *Elettaria cardamomum,* is an essential oil that stimulates and tones the digestive tract and has antiseptic properties that stimulate the phagocytic cellular action of the immune system. It is also supportive of the nervous system and helps supplement healthy oral care with its anti-infectious, antibacterial actions.

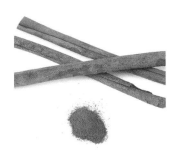

Cinnamon, *Cinnamomum ceylanicum*. Our true cinnamon bark essential oil from Madagascar is antiseptic and antibacterial. It stimulates blood circulation to the gums and promotes their health and regeneration. Cinnamon is high in the compounds *eugenol* and *cineol*, both of which have potent anesthetic and antiseptic properties that increase the production of white blood cells. According to the work of Drs Franchomme and Pènoel, cinnamon bark oil is effective against 98% of all pathogenic bacteria.[27]

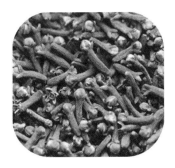

Clove Bud, *Eugenia carophyllata*, is an analgesic essential oil from the flowering buds of the clove tree with an extremely high ORAC. Clove has relieved toothaches and freshened breath since ancient times. A potent antibacterial, antiviral, and antifungal, clove boosts the immune system and stimulates blood flow with its botanical constituents of *eugenol*, *esters*, and *sesquiterpenes*,

---

[27] *L'aromatherapie exactement*. 1990, Roger Jollois Editeur,

all of which combine to create an essence with an impressive action against pathogens and microbes. "It is antiparasitic and helps gum infections, toothaches and tonsillitis."[28]

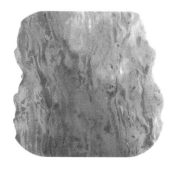

Mastic, *Pistacia lentiscus*, is a type of resin similar to frankincense which comes from the inner sap of the mastic tree and is helpful for maintaining the connective tissue in the oral area. It has a long history of oral care use in ancient Greece and is very good in helping to remove tooth plaque. Mastic contains antioxidants, antifungal, and antibacterial benefits. The major antibacterial components of mastic oil are: *a-Pinene*, *verbenone*, *a-terpineol*, *linalool*, *β-myrcene*, *β-pinene*, *limonene*, and *β-caryophyllene*[29]. Like all essential oils, the antibacterial efficacy of mastic oil is due to all of its components working synergistically. This resin extract is a potent antiseptic, which inhibits oral bacteria including *Helicobacter pylori* that creates stomach ulcers. Mastic oil helps to harness the activity of the blood's first-line-of-defense protection: the leukocytes (white blood cells) and the multinucleocytes. This helps to increase the tissue's defense, especially between the teeth and gums, where gingivitis and plaque occur.

---

[28] *Medical Aromatherapy*, K. Schnaubelt p. 216:1999
[29] Chemical Composition and Antibacterial Activity of the Essential Oil and the Gum of *Pistacia lentiscus*, *J. Agric. Food Chem.*, 2005, 53 (20), pp 7681–7685

Neem, *Azadiracta indica*, has pain-relieving compounds that can reduce the discomfort of a toothache. The vasodilatation and anti-inflammatory

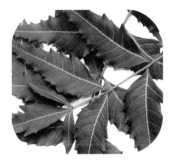

compounds in neem prevent cell adhesion and kill the bacteria that cause tooth decay. Neem alkalizes the gums and mouth, and kills the bacteria that cause *Pyorrhea* and *Gingivitis*. Neem obliterates the calcium-forming organisms and the organisms that cause cavities. Neem is *'arista,'* which in Sanskrit means "perfect, complete, and imperishable." Neem has been used in Ayurvedic traditions for thousands of years in agriculture, food storage, and medicine. Many research studies prove that neem is fungicidal, miticidal, and antibacterial. Neem oil is an ideal remedy to eliminate periodontal and tooth infection. It can be applied locally around the teeth and gums and also benefits the gastrointestinal tract.

Oregano, *Origanum vulgare*, wild oregano oil from

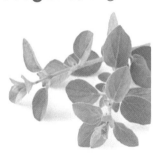

the mountains of the Mediterranean, has a bounty of botanical benefits with a broad spectrum of antibacterial, antifungal, anti-parasitic, anti-microbial, anti-viral, and anti-inflammatory action. Wild oregano contains two phenol compounds (in the following concentrations) that contribute to its medicinal applications: *carvacrol* at over 65% and *thymol* at 3.4%. These phenols possess potent antiseptic, analgesic, and antibacterial properties. Dr. Gerald Smith, DDS, explains, "Basically, oregano works like an antibiotic," boosting the immune system. Many studies show that oregano has a broad range of antimicrobial activities and works against fungus, virus, and bacteria, including *E. coli, Staphylococcus aureus, and Pseudomonas aeruglinosa*. Wild oil of oregano in oral applications can also improve dental hygiene as it destroys plaque-causing bacteria and reduces risks of gum disease.

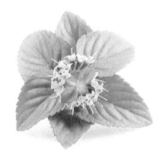

Peppermint, *Mentha piperita*, helps with digestion and has an analgesic and cooling anti-inflammatory effect. Ingesting peppermint oil reduces levels of oxidized fats in body tissue and reverses declines in glutathione that were caused by radiation exposure[30]. Our peppermint is a genuine distillation of the fresh leaves and comes from a fourth generation family of distillers in France. It is important to understand that the peppermint flavouring in commercial toothpaste is artificial menthol and offers no benefit in preventing gingivitis. Real peppermint is a potent anti-oxidant and inhibits the bacterium that causes tooth decay.

---

[30] "Peppermint vs. Radiation Damage", *Journal of Radiation Research*, (Ref. 3) Samarth and Kumar, 2003

Rose Otto, Rosa *damascena,* is an elegant and precious essence. It takes sixty roses to make one

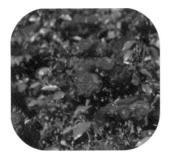

drop of Rose Otto essential oil! One of the most medicinally valued extracts, it adds resiliency and elasticity to the gum tissue. It is an effective analgesic and is *vulnerary,* meaning that it speeds up the healing of tissues with its potent antiviral and antiseptic properties. It is great for cold sores and cankers. Rose Otto also has the ability to regenerate connective tissues and tonify the gums.

Seabuckthorn Berry, *Hippophae rhamnoides,* is an

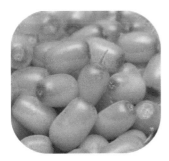

incredibly rich and vital oil; extracted from a berry, it is perfectly balanced in omega 3, 6, 7, and 9 oils. Our seabuckthorn berry is a special super critical extract that is able to capture over 190 bioactive substances from the edible berry. The oil is also potent in antioxidants, anti-inflammatory beta carotene, carotenoids, and phytosterols that reduces redness and helps heal mucous membranes. I have been using seabuckthorn in many of my formulas since 1994 and have found the oil regenerates cells, protects against cell water loss, and is rich in vitamins C, E, and provitamins A and

The Benefits of Botanicals

B's. Seabuckthorn Berry is rich in lipids, beneficial fatty acids, and rare palmitoleic acids. All of these extraordinary plant properties contribute to regenerate and revitalize connective and gingival tissue.

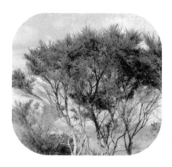

Tea Tree Oil, *Malaleuca alternifolia*, from the paper bark tea tree, has been used for thousands of years as a medicinal plant by the Australian Aborigines. Tea tree oil has anti-viral, anti-fungal, and anti-bacterial properties, and is "A therapeutic agent in chronic gingivitis and periodontitis, conditions that have both bacterial and inflammatory components."[31] Tea tree is very high in natural anti-inflammatory agents and contains the plant-chemicals *cineol* and *propanol*, both kinds of natural chemicals that can decrease gingivitis and reduce plaque. Tea tree also helps stop the approach of bacteria and is very astringent and antiseptic. In a scientific dental study,[32] a genuine distillation of tea tree oil (2.5%) proved effective in the treatment of chronic of gingivitis and inflammation. High in natural anti-inflammatory, antibacterial constituents of 1.8 –cineol, terpinen-4-ol, tea tree essential oil decreased the level of gingival teeth and reduced plaque scores in the study. Furthermore, the study showed that a total of 162 oral bacteria isolates (including streptococcus)

---

[31] *Australian Dental Journal* 2004; 49: (2):78, S. Soukoulis, R. Hirsch.)
[32] Ibid, p.78

were inhibited and rapidly destroyed by tea tree oil concentrations of less than 2%. The study concluded, "The components of Tea Tree Oil are known to have lipophilic properties which facilitate its diffusion through the epithelium. If Tea Tree Oil is readily absorbed after topical application into the gingival tissues and has anti-inflammatory properties once it has entered the connective tissues, it would be a unique non-toxic agent."[33] The *Healthy Gum Drops* formula contains more than 2% of this astringent and antiseptic essence.

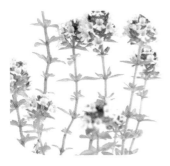

Thyme Linalool, *Thymus officinalis linalool*, is a rare variety of the thyme species. It is both antiseptic and gentle. Thyme Linalool balances oral salivary secretions, stimulates the immune system, and acts as a decongestant. Overall, it is a tonifying and effective immuno-stimulant with anti-bacterial agents.

Essential oils in their unique nature are all antibacterial, antifungal, and antiviral to varying degrees. In the book *Beyond Antibiotics*, Michael Schmidt devotes an entire chapter to the antimicrobial efficacy of essential oils, and states, "One of the advantages essential oils have over antibiotics is that bacteria do not develop resistance to essential oils. Many essential oils exert their antibacterial effect by interfering with the bacteria's ability to breathe. On the other hand, antibiotics interfere with the

---

[33] Ibid, p.83

life cycle, or metabolism of, bacteria, but since bacteria are very crafty creatures, they change their chemistry and genes, which makes the antibiotic less effective the next time it is used. As a result, new generations of antibiotics will need to be developed to stay ahead of these organisms. Additionally says Schmidt, "another advantage to essential oils is that some actually stimulate immune function."[34]

The botanical serums created for the Successful Self-Dentistry protocol are *Healthy Gum Drops* and *Yogi Tooth Serum*. Many people have asked us, "What is the difference between the two and which should I use?" The answer is that they have the same effect and the same excellent results, yet they contain different synergies of botanicals. All the ingredients are active and all the ingredients are antibacterial, antifungal, and antiviral, meaning they can remove unwanted oral bacteria, revivify gum tissue, and enhance the immune system.

Yogi Tooth Serum and *Healthy Gum Drops* achieve the same results with different botanical selections. They maximize the health of one's oral ecology by both rejuvenating the gum tissue and increasing blood circulation to the gums and blood vessels of the mouth. The *Healthy Gum Drops* is fresh and minty tasting. The powerful bitters of neem in *Yogi Tooth Serum* take some people a little getting used to (although the cinnamon and cardamom in the product do help make the neem palatable). That being said, there is no need to get both, although

---

[34] Schmidt, *Beyond Antibiotics: Strategies for Living in a World of Emerging Infections and Antibiotic-Resistant* Bacteria ,2009

some choose both for variety and alternate between the two. Both serums are great for flossing, brushing, and for keeping gums healthy, which is a major key to oral health. Both formulas are also effective on a deeper level and, while they work wonders at cleaning the teeth and nourishing the gum tissue, they are also beneficial to digestion and the stomach. So, even if you are only focusing on the teeth and gums, the botanicals in these serums are part of an integrated, harmonious system that can also benefit your whole body.

People sometimes ask if it is okay if they happen to swallow any of the oral care serums. The short answer is yes, in the "drop" quantities in which they are used. Essential oils are potent and it is often advised they not be taken internally in any quantity. This is true if the oils are not a genuine authentic distillation. However, when pure distillations of essential oils are taken in small quantities (i.e. by the drop), most are fine (and often beneficial) for internal use. In fact, many essential oils are used by the food and flavor industries. Orange juice is often flavoured with essential oil from oranges, Earl Grey Tea is flavoured with essential oil distilled from bergamot, and many liqueurs, confectionaries, chocolates, and flavour extracts use various essential oils. Essential oils are lipid soluble and, because they have a small molecular size, are able to penetrate the dermal layer of the skin, positively affecting the body through the lymphatic vessels, capillaries, cells, and nerve endings located there.

What Goes on the Skin Goes In

Aside from being cautious about what and how much is ingested by swallowing, it is significant to know that everything that is applied to the body, including essential oils, or the manufactured chemicals of perfumes, toothpaste, and synthetic lotions, are also absorbed into the bloodstream, cells, and organs whenever they are applied to the skin, and often to a higher degree than by eating and digesting something. This rate of absorption is even higher inside the mouth and its moist tissues where the skin wall, or epithelium, is only one cell thick. This is especially true if one has bleeding gums where anything in the mouth will have direct access to the bloodstream. We would not want to put anything in, on, or around the body that could not be swallowed. With ingredients, discernment is important.

8. More Teeth Tips

Alignment - The Right Bite

When new fillings are put in or old ones removed, the way your teeth fit together may feel funny, and the occlusion (your bite) may be out of alignment. Improperly aligned teeth can affect the jaw and nerves along the spine, leading to uncomfortable or chronic aches. Please use a dentist that will check (or have an osteopath that works with the dentist) check the vertebrae in the spine and neck and have the vertebrae brought into alignment. This can be done with a massage, an adjustment, or cranial sacral work and will allow for the best bite position.

Alkalinity - Keeping the Body Alkaline

One can test the alkalinity of the saliva and urine with litmus paper (that yellow strip of paper you used to play with in science class). A healthy, nutrient rich diet is vital in achieving alkalinity in the body! Green things like spirulina, chlorella, green veggie juices, and smoothies are all very alkalinizing. So is baking soda and magnesium. Baking Soda may be also be used as a supplement.

Atomic Iodine Mouth Gargle

An immune-boosting mouth gargle can be prepared with the atomic form of iodine. This has rapid bactericidal activity, clears oral thrush, and is beneficial for the thyroid. Simply add one drop to a glass of water. This can be done from every other day to once a week.

Baking Soda (Sodium Bicarbonate)

I used to think baking soda was a strange white substance - now I understand that sodium bicarbonate is actually a major element present in all body fluids and organs in the body. It is found in the saliva, is secreted by our stomachs, and is necessary for digestion. Aluminum free baking soda is perfectly

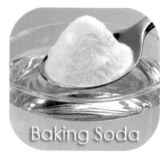

safe to use in the mouth to clean teeth and can even be taken orally to maintain pH levels. Sodium bicarbonate has also been shown to decrease dental plaque acidity, prevent dental carries due to its buffering capacity, and inhibit plaque formation, increase calcium uptake to the enamel, increase the pH of one's oral ecology, and neutralize the effect of harmful metabolic acids. It is also less abrasive to enamel than commercial toothpaste.

Blood Tests

Blood tests can be a wonderful tool for seeing what is going on with the mouth and body. The trick is getting the right professional or doctor to interpret them. Here are some suggestions:

- A general hormone panel: Different hormones are tested for men and women (menstruating women should do their test on day 18-22 to include progesterone levels.)
- C-reactive protein (CPR) and homocysteine levels: This will check the markers of any systemic

inflammation in the body and are a great indicator of general health.

- CBC – Complete Blood Count before and after serious dental procedures to see how the dental material and immune system are getting along.
- Thyroid – TSH levels.
- General vitamins and minerals test - to check for any dietary deficiencies and the body's ability to absorb nutrients.
- For more information on blood tests visit http:// www.lifeextension.com/blood. A blood sugar monitor is easy to purchase at any drug store. Check your fasting blood sugar levels every morning.

Breath

There certainly have been plenty of commercials about the subject of bad breath. Beyond the bad breath that is caused by eating garlic or that is caused by mild plaque that may appear in the morning, if you find your breath is less than fresh after brushing and flossing and you are free of cavities, it may be a message from your body that something needs to be balanced. The source could be sulfur compounds being released from the stomach and/ or old root canals or decay under a crown-filling. The body may be processing a large bacterial load due to inflammation or it may be due to having a dry mouth at night (due to lack of saliva flow from medication, sleep apnea, or snoring). Or one may have to dig deeper and explore digestive issues. The health of the mouth reflects the health of the intestinal tract. Gas, bloating, constipation, and/or high blood sugar could all be root causes of issues with breath. To remedy halitosis, be sure there is no active decay in the mouth and do the 8 Step Successful Self-Dentistry protocol twice a day. Examine your digestive process to see if your body needs enzymes, probiotics, colonics, or clay therapy so that it can come into balance.

Clay

Clay has been used for internal and external purification since ancient times. Either by bathing in clay or packing it on the body, clay has the ability to pull out toxins and heavy metals through the skin. The use of clay packs in the mouth and ingesting clay also works by pulling toxins from the intestinal tract and mouth. When it interacts with the body, clay engages in a dynamic state of ionic exchange with the tissues and the alimentary canal. The adsorption power of bentonite clay, for example, is very effective at pulling toxins into its inner structure. The clay absorbs positively charged toxins and impurities and leaves healthy negatively charged nutrients behind.

Clay is also wonderful for brushing the teeth. For a fine polish, simply sprinkle very fine, powdered clay

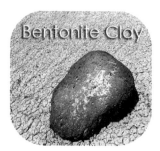
Bentonite Clay

(bentonite, zeolite and/or silica rich clay) onto your dry toothbrush for a polish that will clear up plaque. A clay pack is also helpful for detoxifying the site of a mercury tooth extraction, an abscess, or inflamed gums. Clay packs work by absorbing toxins from deeper layers of the oral tissues. To make a clay pack, combine two drops of *Healthy Gum Drops* or *Yogi Tooth Serum* *with* non-chlorinated, non-fluoridated water and clay to make a little clay ball. Place the clay ball firmly against the affected area of the mouth for ten minutes[35], then discard and rinse with spring water. Good sources for clay are www.vitalityherbsandclay.com and www.magneticclay.com.

Gums - Very Inflamed

This tip was in the "preparing for the dentist" section, and it is so helpful that I am listing it here again. A great tip from Dr. Hal Huggins for very inflamed gums is to thoroughly and vigorously swish salt water around the mouth every hour for two days (half a teaspoon of pure sodium chloride to a glass of warm water) and on the half hour, rinse with *sodium ascorbate* vitamin C powder (this is *not* the acid form of vitamin C ascorbate acid, which is acidic and only has a pH of one). Huggins explains that salt kills the bacteria and Vitamin C creates the electrons (unhealthy tissue is saturated with protons and healthy tissue is saturated with electrons).

Healing Herbs

Herbal tea goes far beyond the tea one makes with little tea bags. David Wolfe says, "The days of teabags are over! Make a big pot of tea, this will

---

[35] If possible, lie down outside and let the sunshine into your mouth while you have your clay pack on, this will further activate its properties.

nourish you." One of my favourite methods of making

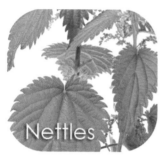

Nettles

herbal tea is to put 1-2 oz of dry herbs into a quart sized (32 oz/1000 ml) Mason jar. Fill the Mason jar with almost boiling water, cap it, and let steep overnight. Strain and drink in the morning. You can fill several jars in this manner and keep them in the fridge after they have had an overnight steep. An overnight infusion of nettles will yield about 500mg of calcium per cup. A **Mineral Rich Tea** with Horsetail, Nettles, and Dandelion is a wonderful tonic for toning the liver, the skin, and the digestive process. It also strengthens tooth enamel and gum tissue. Dandelion brings minerals to the teeth, horsetail is high in silica, and nettles are rich in calcium and iron.

Make an **Herbal Powder Poultice**. Think of this as a spa treatment for your teeth and gums. It is like making a miniature face mask for your mouth. Start by taking one capsule, or a dash, of powdered goldenseal, astralagus, and/or white oak bark and mix with *Yogi Tooth Serum* or *Healthy Gum Drops* until you have a paste. Now pack this mixture into the pockets between the teeth and the areas that

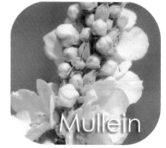

Mullein

need extra care. This can also be combined with clay (please see the Clay section).

Herbal Mouth Rinse – Add herbal tinctures to your 16 oz of salt brine and rinse or put this healing tonic through the vita pik or water pik. Use Mullein, white oak bark, goldenseal, graperoot, and/or ginger.

Heavy Metal Detox

Heavy metals are toxic substances that accumulate in the blood stream and body fat. They are the result of decades of industrialization. A multi-faceted approach is best to gently chelate[36] the body through a combination of herbs, supplements, and therapies. In this day and age, it is good to cleanse, either through a daily practice of dry brushing and sweating in a sauna, for example, or by having a series of colonics once or twice a year. Furthermore, it is necessary to eliminate all synthetic body care "beauty" products and household cleaning products.

Green is good. When Ron (my partner) had his mercury amalgams removed nine years ago, we made him a mix of fresh cilantro[37] juice and chlolorella powder, which he took with R-alpha-

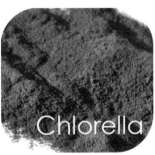

Chlorella

---

[36] Chelation therapy is a process by which toxic substances in the body, in particular metals can be converted to less toxic forms and safely secreted.

[37] Cilantro is an intracellular chelator it mobilizes heavy metals from the central nervous system and other tissues

lipoic acid (R-ALA) capsules. Ron took this combination daily for three months in order to remove any latent heavy metals from his body. Chlolorella, green algae, is able to bind with pesticides, mercury, and other heavy metals and assist with their removal from the body. In his book, *Superfoods*, David Wolfe states, "When chlorella is ingested by the human body, it dramatically increases the rate of rebuilding and healing in tissues, multiplies the growth rate of lactobacillus (beneficial bacteria) in the bowel, boosts the immune system, and fights free-radical damage." It is also worth looking into supplements that support this process: MSM[38], magnesium[39], taurine, probiotics, vitamin C, spirulina, NAC (N-Acetyl-L-Cysteine to boost glutathione levels), zinc, kelp, and selenium. You will also want to support your liver function with turmeric, glutathione, milk thistle, natural B vitamins, and SOD (super oxide dismutase). You can help your bowels[40] detoxify with a tablespoon of chia seeds and a teaspoon of bentonite clay soaked overnight in a glass of water to drink in the morning.

Other treatments:
Far infrared sauna heaters emit a special wavelength designed to release heavy metals through the body's glands. Sweating is a safe and effective way to remove stored toxins, as they are excreted through the skin rather than through the kidneys

---

[38] Methysulfonylmethane (MSM) aids in detoxifying metals by giving sulfur to methionine and cysteine
[39] Healthy magnesium levels lead to safer detoxification and chelation
[40] It is vital to keep healthy elimination flowing to avoid stagnancy and reabsorption.

and the liver, which are taxed by the job. You can dry brush before daily baths, showers, or saunas, as this stimulates the lymph system and is a wonderful longevity practice. Another gentle way to detoxify is through cleansing clay baths, add baking soda and clays to your bathing experience with the addition of a drop of the immune enhancing, lymph stimulating essential oils of juniper, grapefruit, and cypress to enhance your bathing experience.

Homeopathy

Homeopathic remedies are the use of highly diluted substances based on the principle of "like cures like." These remedies are useful tools to help balance one's oral ecology by strengthening, detoxifying, and getting to the root of oral imbalances. Some biological dentists, like Dr. Gerald Smith inject homeopathic remedies[41] into extraction sites and use homeopathics to balance the negative effects of root canals, cavities, and imbalances in the saliva and enamel. Dr. Smith feels that, "If you hit the right remedy for the right problem it will work through mint, coffee, alcohol, anything."[42] Homeopathic therapy is a vast topic and the following suggestions are just the tip of the iceberg. For more in-depth information please consult a homeopath, check the online resource *Homeopathy for Everyone,* and/or read *The Textbook of Dental Homeopathy* by Colin B. Lessell.

Belladonna for abscesses and TMJ

---

[41] Dr. Smith uses *Sanum Remedies* from Germany and combines with Rife Technology

[42] An interview with Dr. Smith with Patrick Timpone on the www. oneradionetwork .com, July 2009

Hypericum for repairing tissue that has been damaged by bacteria
Arnica for any dental work, dental trauma, extractions and/or pain from swelling
Plantago Top tooth ache remedy
Coffea for severe tooth aches that make one feel "crazy"

Tissue Salts/Cell Salts are another form of homeopathic remedy, developed by German physician Dr. Wilhelm Heinrich Schüessler, which is based on inorganic mineral salts. Here are four Cell Salt suggestions that may be useful in your dental apothecary:

Calc Fluor: Indicated for poor tooth enamel, sensitive teeth, decay, and weakened elasticity of tissue. This I have experienced firsthand - after a few passionate weeks of ingesting fresh wild bee pollen, I discovered that, because the bee pollen was slightly acid, it had affected my enamel. Luckily, I ran into my naturopathic doctor friend and found that she had had a similar experience. She advised taking 3-4 tablets of Cal Fluor Cell Salts, swishing them around the mouth with water, and then spitting out. I am happy to report that my enamel was back to normal in three days.

Calc Phos: May help balance calcium/phosphorus ratios in bones. Its primary function is to build solid dentine and enamel. Also used as a remedy for teething; suggested to use with Calc Fluor for decay. Think of Calc Phos for the matrix inside the teeth and Calc Fluor for the external.

Nat Mur (Sodium Chloride): A fluid balancer, it maintains the body's water balance by controlling the movement of water in and out of the cells. Indicated for dry mouth, lack of saliva, cold sores and/or cracked tongue.

Silica: Major constituent of blood, skin, hair, nails, bones, nerve sheaths, and some tissues. Helpful for treatment whenever there is pus formation - for example: abscesses, pus pockets, or gum infection.

Hydrogen Peroxide

Food-grade hydrogen peroxide is the type of peroxide you will want to keep handy. This is the undiluted liquid and it is very strong so it needs to be watered down to a concentration of 3% to use. Use it *once in a while* to flush out a gum pocket or *once a year* to whiten your teeth - rinse immediately with salt water to neutralize and alkalinize. It is too astringent on the enamel and the gums to use every day, and with overuse, one may experience gums pulling back a bit from the astringency. You definitely want to have hydrogen peroxide as part of your tool kit because it is the best solution for cleaning tooth brushes and dental tools. Each member of the family can store their toothbrush in a small glass of 3% hydrogen peroxide solution overnight. Remember to change the solution daily.

Magnesium Oil

Magnesium chloride, in its natural pure form, is helpful in healing and strengthening teeth and tissue. It is essential for proper calcium absorption to form strong enamel and essential mineral for bone matrix. A solution of natural liquid magnesium chloride diluted with water (50:50) is also an excellent mouthwash for revitalizing oral ecology. The purest form can also be swallowed. Use full strength or dilute up to 50% to use as a mouth rinse once a day or once a week, depending on one's oral condition. Dilute for children. Quality magnesium oil can be found at www.longevitywarehouse.com

Oil Pulling Therapy

An ancient Ayurvedic oral care technique to heal bleeding gums, making teeth whiter and freshening less than pleasant breath is to rinse the mouth with a mix of organic virgin coconut oil (or olive oil), one drop of oregano essential oil, and either Healthy Gum Drops or Yogi Tooth Serum. Swish this mix in the mouth daily and vigorously for 10 minutes then spit out. The oil pulls toxins from teeth and gums. For more information, read the book *Oil Pulling Therapy* by Dr. Bruce Fife.

Ozone for Oral Care

Ozone is made of three atoms of oxygen (O3) and has many applications in oral care, as nascent oxygen is naturally antifungal, anti-bacterial, and anti-viral. It was the brilliant visionary, Nikola Tesla, an electrical genius with over 300 patents for a wireless light bulb, wireless communication, ionized gases, cold plasma, and ozone generation for oxygen therapy that invented ozone therapy. In 1896, Tesla was issued a patent for an ozone generator. He formed the *Tesla Ozone Company* and went into production of these generators. He produced a powerful gel made by bubbling ozone through olive oil until it solidified for use by naturopaths and doctors.

Today, biological dental practices use ozone in the form of ozone gas and ozone infused water.

Ozonated gas has many dental uses; among these is the practice of injecting it around the root of a root canalled tooth. Cavities exposed to ozone gas will subsequently harden. In the case of a nerve exposure, ozone water followed by ozone gas will often prevent the nerve from dying. Irrigation of a surgical site with ozone water will speed healing and help remineralize the bone. The gas injected into cavitations sites is part of a protocol to clear up the cavitation. Injection of ozone into the TMJ joint has been found to be anti-inflammatory. Ozonated water is used for ingesting, gargling, and irrigating gum pockets. At home, *Ozonated Tooth Serums* deliver the combined benefits of ozone with potent botanicals and these ozonated gels may be applied to gums, sensitive teeth, abscesses, gum pockets, sulca, mouth lesions, and cold sores.

Salt

Salt is a simple and powerful anti-bacterial alkalinizing agent. Dr. Hal Huggins recommends using only pure sodium chloride (purified salt) over sea salt. He states sea salt may be laden with heavy metals and has lost its electrical charge, and 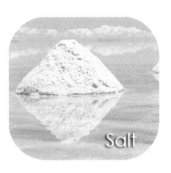 sodium, potassium, and chloride are all involved in an important electrical exchange within the cells of the body. Take the sea salt and dissolve in hot water to recharge the electrons of the sodium and potassium. Sea salt has non-biological potassium in it and is often contaminated with lead, mercury, cadmium, and other heavy metal contaminants.

Stress Less

The key to less stress is *cortisol reduction*. Cortisol is a hormone secreted from over-anxious adrenal glands. When this happens it can lead to adrenal exhaustion, and, with the extra cortisol in the body, can upset the entire hormonal orchestra, creating further stress and imbalance. Though sometimes easier said than done!, de-stressing can be helped with herbs, healthy food choices, eliminating caffeine, yoga, any kind of body movement that makes you sweat, saunas, acupuncture, cranial sacral treatments, meditation, and massage therapies. My favourite way to relieve stress is laughing till my eyes water and walking in nature with my feet touching the ground. An herbal compound of magnolia flower and cork bark, marketed as *Relora* is an effective and non-drowsy way to both reduce cortisol levels and increase levels of the beneficial hormone DHEA. In one study, DHEA was found to reduce cortisol levels by 37% over a two week period.[43] Passionflower decreases anxiety and is good for insomnia as it creates restful sleep. Another helpful stress-less aid is 5HTP, a derivative of the amino acid tryptophan, which helps the body create serotonin and has been found to increase REM sleep.

Teething

Teething can often challenge a baby's immune system and may be accompanied by inflamed

---

[43] http://douglaslabs.com/pdf/pds/98739.pdf

swollen gums, ear infections, colds, diarrhea, and irritability. Raising your little ones intake of phosphorus and vitamin C can be very helpful during teething. Homeopathic remedies of *Camillia* (a homeopathic combination) or single homeopathic remedies of chamomile, belladonna, and pulsatilla are gentle and effective in this area. One drop of essential oil of roman chamomile or lavender diluted with one drop of jojoba and massaged into cheeks and jaw can also relieve discomfort. To calm inflammation, half a drop of organic clove oil diluted in virgin coconut oil, or half a drop of *Wild Child Healthy Gum Drops* can be applied to the gums.

Thyroid Care

"Most plants do not need iodine, but humans require it for the production of thyroid hormones that regulate the metabolic energy of the body and set the basal metabolic rate (BMR)." David Wolfe, *Superfoods*

Many folks experience inefficient thyroid function, often because the thyroid is deeply affected by radiation, heavy metals, and BPA leeching from some plastic fillings. The thyroid is burdened with brominated bread, chlorine showers, fluoride in water, toothpaste and mercury fillings leaking 24/7. Mercury toxicity, even at low levels, can interfere with cell reproduction causing fatigue and lowering body temperature, which in turn makes it difficult for the thyroid to balance. If blood TSH is above 2, this could be an indicator of a heavy metal problem.

Iodine can help remove mercury, fluoride, radiation, and bromide from the body. These heavy metals are often trapped in the thyroid and will affect its function. *Lugols* iodine can be applied transdermally on a daily basis - transdermal application is more efficient because the iodine does not have to pass through the digestive system and liver. If your skin does not retain the colour of the iodine for a couple hours, you may be deficient in iodine.

Thyroid Health - A DVD with Tonic Herbalist Truth Calkins and author David Wolfe
www.longevitywarehouse.com/Thyroid-Health-p/ thyroidhealthset.htm

Toothaches

Toothaches can be excruciating and are a wake-up call from your mouth. A toothache may be caused by a damaged nerve or from bacteria penetrating the enamel or a nerve. For first aid treatment, dilute organic clove or rose otto essential oil to provide both anti-bacterial and analgesic relief. Dilute two drops of clove or rose otto oil in *Yogi* 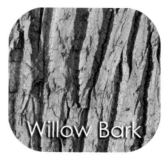 *Tooth Serum*, *Healthy Gum Drops*, organic olive oil, or virgin coconut oil and apply the essential oils to the affected area. Apply every half hour until pain eases. Another option is to dilute the rose or clove oil in a ratio of 1:3 with olive oil and then inject into the gum line or affected area with a vita-pik or a blunt tipped syringe. After this is done, cover the tooth with propolis paste or frankincense resin to create a clean, sealed area. Willow bark herb, the plant that aspirin is derived from, is also very effective. Other helpful toothache herbs that may be taken in liquid tinctures or capsule form include: osha root, ginger, turmeric, mullein, white oak bark, and goldenseal. Interesting research on B12 has also found that unidentified dental pain and neuralgia related to jaw infection can be relieved by the injectable methyl form of vitamin B12. More information and a safe protocol for its use can be found in the appendix of Dr. Manuel Esperanca's book *The Wonders OF Vitamin B12: Keep Sane and Young*. Additionally, the root causes of toothache can be kept at bay by keeping the immune system boosted with extra vitamin C, reishi tincture, vitamin D, chaga tea, olive leaf extract, oil of oregano (dilute wild oregano essential oil to 5% to 95% olive oil), and pine bark extract.

TMJ - The Temporomandibular Joints

The TM joints are on the left and right side of the face and connect the upper and lower jaw. As well, there are 136 muscles attached to the lower jaw. These muscles and joints affect the alignment of the teeth, as well as that of the occipital ridge, the neck and the shoulder girdle, which in turn affects the pelvic girdle and the way one walks. These muscles, along with proprioception[44] and balancing of the upper and lower jaw can be out of alignment due to a number of reasons: including a forceps birth delivery, which, due to pressure on the cranium, can distort alignment, fillings, root canals, extractions, and excessive dental procedures - especially when

---

[44] The unconscious perception of movement and spatial orientation arising from stimuli within the body itself.

teeth have been ground/filed down. If your tongue rests pressing at the roof of your mouth, you may be carrying extra tension in your mouth and jaw. Throughout the day, your tongue should be resting at the bottom of your mouth. Take a moment to feel where your tongue is as you are reading. Also, if you hear a clicking sound when you open and close your mouth, it might be an indication that your TMJ is out of alignment and needs balancing. An unbalanced bite can cause compression in the TM joint leading to headaches, blurred vision near-sightedness[45] and stress. Dr. Weston Price found that when processed foods are eaten in the years of physical growth before 18, the jaw (the maxilla) does not develop properly, which can cause crowding in the mouth and also distort the position of the maxilla (which often leads to wisdom teeth having to be removed). To counter this osteopaths, and craniosacral therapists can gently encourage a realignment of this all important joint, including a rebalancing of the temporal bone, mandible and related soft tissues.

Relaxing the tongue and jaw is of great benefit to those who find themselves clenching and grinding their teeth (bruxism). Teeth clenching can cause gum recession and tiny (imperceptible on an x-ray) fractures from the great force that is applied by the teeth. Nutritionally, phosphorus intake and low blood sugar help with TMJ disorder. Therapies that

---

[45] The eyes are surrounded by muscles and when these muscles get tense, the shorten causing less than perfect vision. To learn about healing and restoring eyesight, I appreciate the books *The Art of Seeing* by Aldous Huxley and *Take of Your Glasses and See* by Jacob Liberman

will also help TMJ are: intra-oral massage from a registered massage therapist (this will adjust the tight oral muscles and may relax them so much you may find yourself leaving your appointment with your jaw hanging open, in a good way!), cranialsacral treatment, a visit to an osteopath, or a good chiropractic adjustment. Another effective way to relax and release tension from the jaw (and from the temples and back of the neck) is to apply essential oil of peppermint, chamomile, lavender, or marjoram to the tight spots and temples. Also, listening to binaural beats or paraliminal audio programs for deep relaxation before bed creates the healing theta brainwaves (theta being the most healing and restorative state of being) that will relax jaw muscles and keep healthy cells humming. Some of my favorite sources for generating theta brainwaves are:

www.learningstrategies.com/Paraliminal/Home.asp
www.brainwave-sync.com/mp3s-theta-frequency-c-12_3.html
www.centerpointe.com

For a soft inexpensive dental tooth guard to protect teeth at night from clenching:
www.totalgard.com

Stretching the jaw, opening the jaw, very, very, very slowly and then breathing deeply with the jaw open 3-5 times per day slowly strengthens and realigns the joints and relaxes the tongue. The Feldenkrais Movement Institute (somatic movement to reduce pain or limitations in movement, and promote general well-being) has released these lessons that help those with TMJ break the cycle of pain and retrain their muscles to support a functionally healthy jaw:

www.tmj-lessons.com/index.html

Vitamins & Supplements for Oral Care – Top Picks

- **R-Alpha Lipoic Acid** (R-ALA) is a fatty acid found in every cell of the body. It is also a double duty metabolic antioxidant that is both a hydrophilic and a lipophilic molecule with the ability to neutralize free radicals in water, blood, and fats. ALA works on the cellular level to produce energy for the mitochondria. It boosts and recycles other antioxidants including vitamin C, vitamin E, and glutathione.

- **N-Acetyl-L-Cysteine** (NAC) is a derivative and bio-available form of the non-essential amino acid cysteine. NAC boosts glutathione levels and is a very effective nutritional supplement - "it performs as a detoxifying agent, anti-doting more toxins than any other substance in the body – even Vitamin C cannot match its antidotal range"[46].

- Lipospheric **Vitamin C** is the most bio-available; Vitamin C also boosts glutathione levels, and is great for collagen and blood vessels. Eat Vitamin

Amla Berries

---

[46] *The Healing Nutrients Within*, Eric R. Braverman, MD, p. 108: 2003

C naturally from organic superfoods like camu camu berry and amla berry.

- Transdermal **Iodine** - Applied to skin for absorption, if the skin does not retain the colour of the iodine for a couple hours, one may be deficient.

- Create **calcium** in the body with dietary **minerals** magnesium, silica and phosphorous (and vitamins D3 and K2). Great sources are leafy greens, spirulina, chia seeds, horsetail herb, and nettles. One should avoid taking calcium supplements - aside from being derived from chalk and often synthetic, they are non bio-available and create excess calcium secretions in the saliva and calcification in the body.

- **Coenzyme Q10** in ubiquinol form is a potent antioxidant that repairs gum tissue and bone matrix.

- Fat-soluble **vitamin D3** is a steroidal precursor hormone (not a vitamin) and is created mainly by our skin being exposed to sunlight. It is great to get 10 minutes a day! In the winter months, one may need to supplement with capsules of 5,000 or 10,000 IU per day depending on skin type and geographical location.

- **Glutathione** (GSH) - all cells on this planet contain glutathione. It is an intracellular antioxidant and tripeptide that is essential for immune function. GSH is known for its ability to protect and detoxify the body.

- Fat-soluble **vitamin K2** is a very important and rare vitamin (Vitamin K1 is found in a variety of leafy green vegetables like kale, parsley, and coriander). Dr. Weston Price found the highest source of K2 is from June grass-fed cow butter or ghee. Liquid Vitamin K2 and K2 supplements made from cultured fermented soy, *natto* are also available. Greenerpastures.org has a fermented, ethically-produced June-grass butter and cod-liver oil in vegetarian capsules. There is also a grass fed ghee (clarified butter) made in a rhythmic cycle with the full and waxing moon from www.pureindianfoods.com.

- Look for vitamins and supplements that are of high quality, from natural sources, and free of excipients like magnesium stearate.

Water

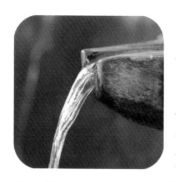

Fresh spring water is the best for your body. Reverse osmosis water may be clean, yet it is also stripped of life-giving minerals, which in turn may leech minerals from your body. Both fluoride and chlorine in tap water are destructive to the teeth. You must always hydrate! Continued dehydration inhibits the saliva from properly lubricating the teeth. To find a spring in your local area, visit www.findaspring.com

9. Further Reading & Resources

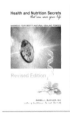 *Health and Nutrition Secrets that Can Save Your Life*, Russell L. Blaylock, MD

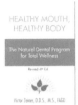 *Healthy Mouth, Healthy Body*, Victor Zeines, DDS

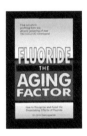 *Fluoride the Aging Factor: How to Recognize and Avoid the Devastating Effects of Fluoride*, John Yiamouyiannis

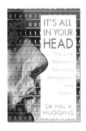 *It's All in Your Head*, Hal Huggins

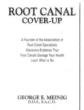

Root Canal Cover-Up, George E. Meinig DDS, FACD

Good Teeth from Birth to Death, Dr. Gerad F. Judd
TMJ Therapy, Robert Peshek, DDS

Concerned father Ramiel Nagel, worried about his daughter's cavities, wrote *How to Cure Tooth Decay* bringing forth much nutritional information to today's times.

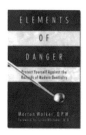

Elements of Danger: Protect Yourself from the Hazards of Modern Dentistry, Morton, D.P.M Walker

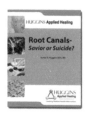

Root Canal: Savior or Sucide, Hal Huggins

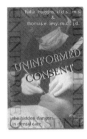

Uninformed Consent, Hal Huggins

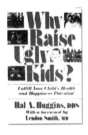

Why Raise Ugly Kids, Hal Huggins

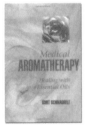

One of my favorite books on the medicinal aspects of aromatherapy is *Medical Aromatherapy*, Dr. Kurt Schnaubelt

A Practical Guide to the Management of the Teeth; Comprising a Discovery of the Origin of Caries, or Decay of the Teeth, with its Prevention and Cure, Parmly, Levi Spear; Free download of this book written in 1819: http://www.archive.org/details/practicalguideto00parm

Websites for Mavericks

Dr. Bob Marshall's making the right dental choices:
www.qnhshop.com/images/QNH/dental/
Making%20the%20Right%20Dental.pdf

Dr. Hal Huggins:
www.terifinfo.com
www.holisticdental.org/
www.hugginsappliedhealing.com/

Audio interviews Nadine has given on oral care (and more):
www.livinglibations.com/media-information

Dr. Gerald Smith:
www.dentalwholebodyconnection.com

Weston Price Foundation:
www.westonaprice.org/component/finder/
search?q=dental

Many of Melvin Page's books can be found on the site for International Foundation for Nutrition & Health: www.ifnh.org

Great interviews in the archives of One Radio Network:
www.oneradionetwork.com/blogcategory/dental_
healing/

Product Resources

Food Grade Hydrogen Peroxide
www.sproutmaster.com

Find a fresh water spring near you

www.findaspring.com

Zappers, clays, magnesium, iodine, MSM, herbs, supplements
www.longevitywarehouse.com

Non-Synthetic Heavy Metal Chelation
http://www.scienceformulas.com

Living Libations Successful Self-Dentistry Serums and Products for healthy teeth and gums available at:
www.livinglibations.com
www.livingearthbeauty.com
www.longevitywarehouse.com
www.surthrival.com
www.therawfoodworld.com

Find a Holistic Biological Dentist
This is a starting point, please interview each dental office
www.greenpeople.org/HolisticDentistry.html
www.holisticdental.org
www.dentalwellness4u.com/freeservices/find_dentists.html
www.iabdm.org/cms/index.php?id=34
www.iaomt.org/patients/search.aspx
www.hugginsappliedhealing.com
www.naturaldentistry.org/referrals_natural_dentistry.htm
www.toxicteeth.org/dentistsDoctorsProducts.cfm
www.toothconservingdentistry.com/p-findadds.html
www.biodentalstudios.com/

Holistic Orthodontists, Cranial Alignment & Bite Specialists

www.aacfp.org/referral.html

www.aago.com/ www.orthotropics.com/

www.cranialacademy.com/search.html?Submit=Accept

www.sorsi.com/locate-doctor

www.cranio.com/directory

www.icnr.com/OrthodonticRelapse.html

www.dentalwholebodyconnection.com

www.amstraussdds.com/

Mercury Information

Dental Amalgam Mercury Syndrome

www.dams.cc

Mercury and its role in Autism and Alzheimer's disease

www.nomercury.org

"Someday, hopefully soon, the dental profession will become extinct... it will happen as soon as the public learns about the cause and cure of cavities and gum problems. No one I've ever known in over 30 years has not wanted to solve their own problems... once they know how."

Dr. Robert O. Nara, D.D.S

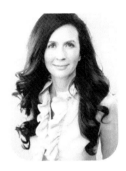

About the Author

Nadine Artemis is the creator of Living Libations, an exquisite line of serums, elixirs and essentials oils for those seeking the purest of the pure botanical health and beauty products on the planet. She is a frequent commentator on health and beauty for media outlets and her products have received rave reviews in *The New York Times*, *The National Post* and *The Hollywood Reporter*. Described by Alanis Morissette as "a true-sense visionary", Nadine has formulated a stunning collection of rare and special botanical compounds. An innovative aromacologist, Nadine develops immune enhancing formulas and medicinal blends for health and wellness: her potent dental serums are used worldwide and provide the purest oral care available. Her healing creations, along with her concept of "Renegade Beauty", encourage effortlessness, eschew regimes and inspire people to rethink conventional notions of beauty and wellness. Nadine's fresh paradigm for beauty and her natural approach to health presents a revolutionary vision: it allows the life-force of flowers, dewdrops, plants, sun, and water to be the ingredients of healthy living and lets everything unessential, contrived, and artificial fall away.

Stay in Touch

Website www.livinglibations.com
Twitter livinglibations
www.facebook.com/livinglibations
www.facebook.com/nadineartemis
www.facebook.com/SuccessfulSelfDentistry

CPSIA information can be obtained
at www.ICGtesting.com
Printed in the USA
249676LV00001B